THE HANDBOOK
NURSE ASSOCIATES
& ASSISTANT
PRACTITIONERS

Sara Miller McCune founded SAGE Publishing in 1965 to support the dissemination of usable knowledge and educate a global community. SAGE publishes more than 1000 journals and over 800 new books each year, spanning a wide range of subject areas. Our growing selection of library products includes archives, data, case studies and video. SAGE remains majority owned by our founder and after her lifetime will become owned by a charitable trust that secures the company's continued independence.

Los Angeles | London | New Delhi | Singapore | Washington DC | Melbourne

THE HANDBOOK FOR
NURSE ASSOCIATES
& ASSISTANT
PRACTITIONERS

GILLIAN ROWE, CHRIS COUNIHAN, SCOTT ELLIS,
DEBORAH GEE, KEVIN GRAHAM, MICHELLE HENDERSON,
JANETTE BARNES & JADE CARTER-BENNETT

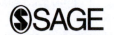

Los Angeles | London | New Delhi
Singapore | Washington DC | Melbourne

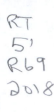

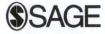
SAGE

Los Angeles | London | New Delhi
Singapore | Washington DC | Melbourne

SAGE Publications Ltd
1 Oliver's Yard
55 City Road
London EC1Y 1SP

SAGE Publications Inc.
2455 Teller Road
Thousand Oaks, California 91320

SAGE Publications India Pvt Ltd
B 1/I 1 Mohan Cooperative Industrial Area
Mathura Road
New Delhi 110 044

SAGE Publications Asia-Pacific Pte Ltd
3 Church Street
#10-04 Samsung Hub
Singapore 049483

Editor: Becky Taylor
Assistant editor: Charlène Burin
Production editor: Katie Forsythe
Copyeditor: Elaine Leek
Proofreader: Christine Bitten
Indexer: Adam Pozner
Marketing manager: Tamara Navaratnam
Cover design: Wendy Scott
Typeset by: C&M Digitals (P) Ltd, Chennai, India
Printed in the UK

Library of Congress Control Number: 2017936481

British Library Cataloguing in Publication data

A catalogue record for this book is available from
the British Library

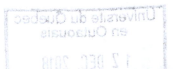
ISBN 978-1-5264-0582-1
ISBN 978-1-5264-0583-8 (pbk)

At SAGE we take sustainability seriously. Most of our products are printed in the UK using FSC papers and boards.
When we print overseas we ensure sustainable papers are used as measured by the PREPS grading system.
We undertake an annual audit to monitor our sustainability.

CONTENTS

LIST OF TABLES AND FIGURES

TABLES

FIGURES

ABOUT THE AUTHORS

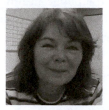 **Gillian Rowe** has edited and authored several chapters of this book. Gillian has extensive experience of the healthcare sector, having been a qualified nurse and then managed a large residential care facility, then lecturing for Plymouth University partnership colleges. Gillian has engaged with the local health community delivering clinical skills training as part of the government's 'Preventing unnecessary admissions' initiative, and has delivered mental health training to the police and armed forces. Gillian is an Associate Fellow of the Higher Education Academy (AFHEA).

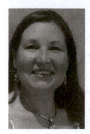 **Janette Barnes** completed her Social Work degree in 2009, and worked for Barnardo's in a project supporting children with disabilities and their families. Much of the work she did centred around families coping with the realisation that their child had a disability and supporting them to gain an understanding of their child's needs. Many of the children were diagnosed with autism – a subject she became fascinated with and has continued to research and advise on. Janette has a teaching qualification and delivers training on disability issues and autism; she has continued to build on her knowledge and experience over the years and enjoys sharing this with others. She also supports and mentors Social Work students. Janette currently works for a Fostering and Adoption Agency.

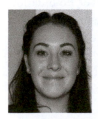 **Jade Carter-Bennett** has been a qualified social worker since 2015, after receiving her BA Hons Social Work degree from Plymouth University. Since then, she has worked within the Adult Social Care sector, specifically with vulnerable adults under 65, which includes young people transitioning from Children's Services. Through this sector, Jade has become involved in work with parents with learning disabilities, something she has a passion for within her work. Prior to becoming a social worker, Jade volunteered for many years at her local Childrens Centre and became an advocate for parents and founder of a parent forum within her community.

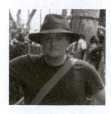 **Dr Chris Counihan** is a Research Associate at Newcastle University. He is a published author and contributor to academic books and journals. He lectures on a range of education and childhood studies programmes at undergraduate and postgraduate levels. His main research interests are how peer-learning networks can accelerate literacy achievement for children from poor backgrounds

and researching education initiatives for gifted and talented children in the developing world. Such interests have taken him to Ghana, Sierra Leone, India and Tanzania
working on various private and UK government projects in capacity-building within the
Education for All and Sustainable Development Goal agendas.

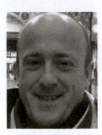

Scott Ellis is a doctoral candidate and lectures at the University of
East London. He has a wealth of experience in the public health
and social care sectors and specialises in research on sexual health
and marginalised groups. He is also an NHS inspector for the Care
Quality Commission and contributes to the NHS National Institute
of Health Research. Scott is a Fellow of the Higher Education
Academy (FHEA).

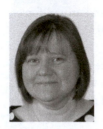

Deborah Gee is a qualified nurse. She has experience in working as a
Specialist Community Public Health Nurse – Health Visitor, including
supporting families and children, offering parenting advice, assessment
of physical and developmental progress, offering advice to the family
when promoting their health and wellbeing in addition to the assessment and identification of health needs of the wider population. With
this experience and her skills and knowledge gained within her PGDip
SCPHN in Health Visiting, BSc (Hons) in Nursing Studies Adult and an MSc in Health
Visiting Biography, she is currently clinical practice educator for Newcastle NHS Trust
and is part of the Northumbria University/Newcastle NHS Trust 'fast track' pilot project.

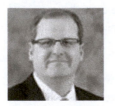

Kevin Graham is a Programme Leader in Higher Education and
has taught a variety of subjects over the years, including Health and
Social Care, Children and Young People's studies, Law, and elements of Sociology at a number of colleges at A-Level, Foundation
Degree and Honours Degree level in the North-East region. Kevin
is also a published author and has previously worked in a variety of
different roles and settings, including managing an educational charity for adults with
learning difficulties, being a Local Authority Cabinet Member for Adult Social Care
and has been an assistant to the former Cabinet Minister for Social Inclusion.

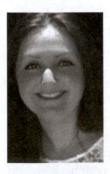

Michelle Henderson has been qualified as a nurse since 2004, having
completed her first degree at Northumbria University. She has worked
in a range of NHS clinical specialties and has also worked in Youth
Offending Services and the Territorial Army. She has worked as a Sister
in Occupational Health, completing a Specialist Community Public
Health Nurse degree at Teesside University. At present, she works
at Public Health England and is completing an MSc in Healthcare
Leadership. Her interests are promoting social mobility, leadership
development and education in the caring professions and public health.

ACKNOWLEDGEMENTS

The authors wish to express their very great appreciation to Becky Taylor and Charlène Burin at SAGE for their help, advice and guidance.

We would also like to give our love, thanks and apologies to our partners, families and friends for their amazing support during the writing process. We really could not have done it without you.

Especial thanks to Johnny and Becci, grammarian extraordinaire, for proofreading.

Further thanks must go to Kerry-Anne Blewitt-Harris and Nichole Anderson, our student reviewers, and Rachael Morice, HE programme leader, whose feedback was invaluable.

Our especial thanks go to Lewis Wade for his amazing drawings.

We are particularly grateful to Dolores Campanario at the World Health Organization for her help with WHO authorised images. Also, many thanks to the following for their amazing support in granting us use of their images: Krishna Stone at GMHC.org, Teri Christenson at Drugfree.org, Marc van Gurp at Osocio.org, Thelma Simmons at communityhealth.ku.edu, Ford Higson at Ishtm.ac.uk, Brian Chittock at aidsvancouver.org, Alan Davidson at the Better Life Chances Unit, Scottish Government, and more thanks to Charlène Burin at Sage for access to the Sage image library.

PUBLISHER'S ACKNOWLEDGEMENTS

Lewis Wade is acknowledged as the original illustrator for the cartoon drawings which appear throughout the book.

ABOUT THE BOOK

In choosing to study as a higher level Healthcare Practitioner, Nurse Associate or to enter into a Nursing Apprenticeship you are following a career choice made since the role was officially created by the NHS and Community Care Act 1990 and the Shape of Caring Review in 2015. The recorded history of caring goes back to the ancient Greeks and Egyptians, and Ayurvedic practitioners have an equally long history. In Christian countries, caring was provided by monks and nuns, and we still call female ward managers 'Sister' as a result of this. Nursing auxiliaries followed Florence Nightingale to the Crimean War (1854–56) but it took until 1955 for the auxiliary role to be formalised. After the 1990 Act, the auxiliary role within the NHS was renamed 'Healthcare Assistant' (HCA).

'Agenda for Change' was introduced in 2002 and it is the NHS career (pay and grading) framework which replaced the old Whitley scale. Implemented in 2004 and, after the Wanless Review (2002) and Francis Report (2013), amended in 2013, it introduced band 4 roles for HCAs. The Cavendish Review (2013) explains that the NHS treats HCAs and the registered nurses who supervise them as separate workforces. Cavendish continued stating that 'A glaring example is the failure to consider how the move to all-degree nursing would affect the career prospects of HCAs. Good hospitals and care homes are now unable to promote some of their best assistants into nursing. This is a waste of talent which must be overcome by urgently developing new bridging programmes.' Higher level care workers and band 4 HCPs/HCAs deserve a career progression and some form of recognition for the work they do, and the new Nurse Associate role goes some way to meeting that recognition.

There has been much debate originating from the Francis Report (2013) regarding training and registration of HCPs/HCAs. Registered nurses have (until now) been responsible for the actions (and inactions) of HCPs/HCAs and this has led to tension around HCPs/HCAs engaging in devolved nursing duties and clinical roles. With the creation of the Nurse Associate (NA) role, comes the creation of a regulatory body under the auspices of the Nursing and Midwifery Council (NMC). It is long overdue.

This book has been constructed by considering the learning dimensions for the Nurse Associate training programme and many aspects of the Nursing Apprenticeship and Foundation Degrees in Health and Social Care and Healthcare Practice. We hope you find it a useful addition to your library.

LEARNING FEATURES: ENGAGING WITH THE TEXT

The book has pedagogic content for you to use as aids to learning, Go Further readings, links to websites and journal articles and reflective activities. These have been designed to stretch and challenge you and deepen your knowledge. This will also help you to become an active independent learner.

Icons

Throughout the book you will see icons in the margin for 'Values', 'Communication and Interpersonal Skills', 'Chapter Cross-references' and 'Person-centred Approach'. These flag up places where these skills are highlighted to support you to deliver high quality care.

Values

Communication & interpersonal skills

Chapter Cross-references

Person-centred Approach

A note on terminology: How are they known?

Throughout this book, those for whom we care are called 'patients'. This is because it is too unwieldy to write 'patient slash client slash service user' each time they are mentioned. So please mentally insert the name you use at your work setting, and we apologise if it gets annoying.

REFERENCES

Cavendish, C. (2013) *Review of Healthcare Assistants and Support Workers in NHS and Social Care*. London: Department of Health. Available at: www.gov.uk/government/publications/review-of-healthcare-assistants-and-support-workers-in-nhs-and-social-care (accessed 18 May 2017).

Francis, R. (2013) *Report of the Mid Staffordshire NHS Foundation Trust Public Inquiry*. London: Stationery Office. Available at: http://webarchive.nationalarchives.gov.uk/20150407084003/http://www.midstaffspublicinquiry.com/report (accessed 10 April 2017).

Wanless, D. (2002) *Securing Our Future Health: Taking a Long-term View*. London: HM Treasury. Available at: http://webarchive.nationalarchives.gov.uk/20130107105354/http://www.hm-treasury.gov.uk/consult_wanless_final.htm (accessed 10 April 2017).

PART ONE

ACADEMIC, PERSONAL AND PROFESSIONAL DEVELOPMENT

1

DEVELOPING ACADEMIC STUDY SKILLS: TECHNIQUES AND GUIDANCE FOR UNDERGRADUATE STUDENTS

Chris Counihan

> Question everything – identify any assumptions that may have been made including the author's stance and what an opposing argument may be; whether there is enough evidence to justify their conclusions and investigate alternative views.
>
> Julie Greenslade, BA (Hons) Student

This chapter will introduce you to the skill set needed to succeed as a higher level student, through using the internet to engage in research, how to sift through the research to locate the information you need and then how to use the information gained properly and to reference it to Harvard convention.

 Glossary

- **HE** Higher education
- **Referencing** Ensuring that you do not commit plagiarism
- **Reflection** The deliberate consideration of troubling thoughts
- **Theory** A hypothesis that has been tested and a theory formulated

INTRODUCTION

This chapter provides a snapshot of various techniques, skills and concepts required for enhancing quality learning outputs in higher education (HE). Each section contains guidance, review and practice examples for transfer into your own study domain. In the first section, we consider how previously acquired skills can be useful in a variety of HE learning situations. Second, we look at how to conduct effective searches online to maximise your time spent analysing, critiquing and producing. Finally, we revisit practical concepts of referencing works in your assignments. Use this chapter as your mini support guide at the beginning or during your course of study.

PREPARING TO LEARN IN HIGHER EDUCATION

It might seem a little odd, but the best way to learn is to revisit skills you already possess. For example, let's say you can speak a second language but your learning goal is to master how to write it. In this case, you look at what you have already understood about the language and build a plan for learning how to write it. Understanding the tools for the job through problem solving, personal reflection and development are essential to your success in HE. Recognition for prior learning is key for you plans as you take previously acquired skills and implement them into future learning activities.

One of the problems when we think about learning, is the relationship it has with schooling, which may lead to the resurfacing of old nightmares and panic-stricken worry. I include myself in this. You might reflect on a disastrous learning journey; moreover, you might feel unrewarded or unchallenged – hence your interest now in studying for a degree. Lots of neurological research has your back here. When threatened, our brains go into shutdown. The amygdala, which is in the centre of our brains, is trained in the art of detecting stressful events and determining whether you turn into a Persian Kitten, like me, or a Spartan Warrior, roar!

Fortunately, learning has changed and HE offers open forums to include discussion, debate and personal reflection, thus enabling you to make your own mind up. One of its strengths is the desire to recognise skills and use them in a variety of academic contexts. We might consider academic reading, writing and presenting ideas as being too challenging, but we all have skills that we can use for academic study. The truth is, we use most of these unconsciously every day, which makes them perfect to be developed for academic study.

You already possess remarkable abilities for making analytical, creative and practical judgements. Consider when buying an item of clothing, you analyse the price, shape and colour. Perhaps you will compare it with another piece of clothing before making a decision. Furthermore, being creative doesn't necessarily mean you will build a robot that writes essays; instead, you will deploy solutions based on personal and professional experiences. Finally, being practical, here you will draw upon skills that have not been taught to you, things you are able to do naturally without pause for thought. Recognise when you can select one (or more) of your superpowers when approaching learning in the HE environment. You may be pleasantly surprised at how well they will serve you. Learning to use your intellectual faculties, such as asking questions of the texts you are reading, is a skill that you will need to develop. Table 1.1 gives you guidance.

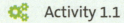 Activity 1.1

Using Sternberg's triarchic model of intelligence, reflect on your own learning and work experiences, then write down one example for each.

Robert Sternberg (1985) has researched intelligence all around the world. He views intelligence in his 'triarchic model', which includes the following three classifications.

Table 1.1 Using your intelligence

Analytical	Creative	Practical
Intellectual capability to problem solve, complete tests and make informed judgements	Intellectual capability to tackle unusual problems drawing on pre-existing skills and experiences – the 'thinking outside of the box' approach to problems	Intellectual capability to deploy 'tacit' skills to a unique set of problems. There might not be an exam, course or guidance for such a scenario and it depends on your interaction with the experience first hand

DEVELOPING SKILLS AND TECHNIQUES FOR ONLINE SEARCHES

Let's look at some of the basic skills. When researching a topic, it is vital that you are able to locate information required to fulfil assessment criteria. The following five tips will demonstrate how to effectively navigate along the information highway:

1. **Control 'F'** – The Time Saver! It operates a mini-search function within any web page, article and/or other word processing software. It works by pressing the 'Control' button (Command button if you are using a Mac) followed by the 'F' button on your keyboard. From here, a box will appear in the top right of the browser. Typing any word into the box and pressing return will automatically search the entire document for your chosen word. This command can be particularly useful if you are reviewing/searching an article for predetermined keywords.
2. **BOOLEAN** searches can enable a specific focus for a key word and term searches. Type in the following commands separately to narrow down searches:
    a. OR – you might want to search for two separate terms such as 'NHS OR Private' – the OR function will list the number of sites that relate to the first or second term
    b. You can combine your searches using phrase and key terms in parenthesis, such as 'Obesity treatment (NHS OR Private)' which will list sites that relate to 'Obesity treatment' on sites containing the words 'NHS' and 'Private', separately

    c.   BUT – this allows terms to be specified while limiting other possible connections. For example, 'Skin cancer BUT NOT melanoma'. Searches will eliminate sites containing 'melanoma' skin cancers and concentrate on listings of non-melanoma hits

    d.   ADJ – this command will look for a term that is positioned within a specified distance (number of words). For example, say you search for 'Public Health obesity ADJ 4'. The search will retrieve all records of 'public' 'health' 'obesity' within 4 words of each other

    e.   Google Advanced Search provides a variety of variables (language, date, region, etc.) for searches and can be found at: www.google.com/advanced_search

3.   **Authority** – Published work and material found online comes in a variety of forms, such as traditional academic articles found in journals, newspapers, magazines, blogs and the like. When considering authority in your searches, you must make a judgement on information presented to you. You should ask yourself the following questions:

    a.   Who is the author and how are they the expert?

    b.   Has it been verified by academic peers (known as peer review)?

    c.   How do I know that it isn't made up?

4.   **Evidence** – It's all about the evidence. It is vital to question everything, unleashing your analytical and evaluative reasoning skills. This means that you must analyse a number of sources before using information in your assignments. Ask the following questions:

    a.   Is the information from opinion or based on studied research material?

    b.   Is there similar evidence that verifies the original claim(s)? Are there other studies, ideas or information that say the same thing?

    c.   Does the article offer a balanced view, that is, the inclusion of counter evidence?

5.   **Time** – As with most things, there is a shelf life. Fortunately, web pages don't smell bad when they go off. The truth is that web pages don't really go off at all, instead, they go into hiding and then reappear when something triggers an associated interest. Fans and users of Twitter will be familiar with trending media; this is essentially the same process. A web page might trend again and accelerate to a higher ranking along the information highway. As Google ranked it highly, you assume that the information is current and decide to use it in your assignment. WARNING! You must investigate the publication date as the web page might have resurfaced from years past and be outdated. You will need to check the date of the original source before employing sentences like these in your work:

    a.   Recent evidence suggests …

    b.   The latest statistics show …

How far back should one go? There's no consensus on this, but as with the terms above – recent and latest – there is an assumption that information is current or is the leading frame of thought at that time. Of course, if your assignment asks that you include historical accounts then you have the licence to trace longer developments, but keep these focused. Seminal theories, famous debates/arguments and other historical content should form the basis of your enquiry.

ASSESSMENTS AND THE APPLICATION OF ANALYTICAL, CRITICAL AND EVALUATIVE REASONING

Understanding assessments

When developing degree level programmes within HE, course leaders have a wealth of assessment methods in their arsenal to choose from. Course leaders will select assessments based on overall module objectives and the inter-disciplinary skills students are required to demonstrate. What is important to understand is that your degree programme is designed specially to accelerate your personal, professional and academic skills and knowledge. Well-planned modules include a broad range of skills and relative assessment methods for subsequent demonstration.

Nightingale et al. (1996) originally suggested eight learning outcomes demonstrable while studying in HE. They include the following:

- Thinking critically and making judgements
- Problem solving and developing plans
- Performing procedures and demonstrating techniques
- Managing and developing oneself
- Accessing and managing information
- Demonstrating knowledge and understanding
- Designing, creating and performing
- Communicating

 Activity 1.2

Write down one example for each of the eight learning outcomes that you have demonstrated in the work or school environment. Include a short description of what and how you did it.

As you can see from Nightingale et al. (1996), there are broad learning outcomes with some interconnections (i.e., communicating and performing) while others are diverse (critical thinking vs. creative outputs). The point is, your degree will encompass each one through a range of skill/vocational assessment methods. But which methods are suitable against each competency? Figure 1.1 provides a synthesis of Nightingale et al.'s (1996) taxonomy and provides details on the types of assessments used against grouped skills.

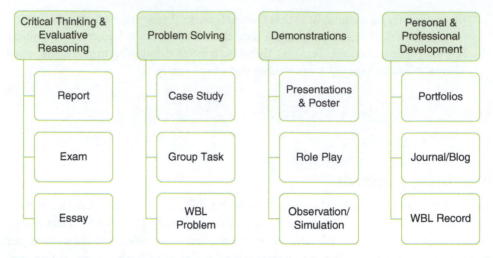

Figure 1.1   Grouped skills and assessment methods

Figure 1.1 is by no means an exhaustive list of core competencies or definite assessments. Instead, it provides a snapshot of the skills/vocational competencies allied to assessment methods that you are likely to face. Course leaders will consider the broader spectrum, so, immediate tasks relate to module assessment tasks, tracking your development across the degree programme.

Essays

Essays are perhaps the most common assessment type in HE. They can vary in length and require time for researching themes, sorting notes, creating arguments and summarising main points. Essays are intended to inform your lecturers as to how well you have understood salient theories, arguments and themes about a studied topic. Let's consider the following essay question from a Healthcare Practice course:

> Justify what is meant by quality of care? Critically appraise the theoretical dimensions of organisational cultures in a chosen UK healthcare provider

To approach the question, it is easier to break down what it is asking us to present for assessment. We can do this in a variety of ways. Firstly, we recognise the keywords, which are usually the verbs as they ask us to do something. In the question above, we note the following verbs and their meaning as:

- Justify – to provide evidence for a claim in knowledge
- Appraise – to evaluate the quality of something through assessing its worth

We use the terminology to help navigate our research about the topic and start to plan the structure of our essay. For the question above, we might adopt the following structure:

Introduction

- To outline how the essay is structured – signposting to core themes such as key policy care documents and legislation. We might consider introducing specific theories that will be referred to, and the organisation chosen as our case study. Essay introductions should offer a sequence to improve the transitions between themes, concepts and major ideas

Middle paragraphs

- Definitions and legal representations of quality of care from a UK perspective
- Salient arguments and key academic debates on future directions of quality of care
- Description of chosen healthcare provider and how they implement/challenge the above (using your placement as a physical reference)
- Examine chosen provider by linking theory to practice in relation to organisational culture

Conclusion

- A summary of the main findings and themes throughout the essay. This will include a brief recap of how you answered the essay question followed by concluding remarks. No new ideas or theories should be introduced here, only a summary of what was investigated and interpreted through your careful analysis

Essay questions and learning outcomes/objectives arrive in various formats. Module guides illustrate what is required for assessment and these will be indispensable when you start to plan your essay. Below are some of the common directive terms, as adapted from Lewis' (1999: 42) comprehensive list of words (and associated meanings) used in essay questioning:

- Analyse – look at multiple parts of something (theme, argument, idea) and examine each in detail
- Describe – provide a detailed account of your subject/topic – usually, answers the what of something
- Discuss – investigate various accounts of something – multiple views or using various arguments giving reasons for each angle
- Compare – look for similarities and differences of something
- Explain – an interpretation followed by an accurate account of something
- Evaluate – supported by valid evidence, an appraisal of something which might include your own reflections (if related to work placement or learning journeys)
- Identify – recognise an important part of something and include brief descriptions
- Interpret – understanding the reality of something, making clear and informed judgements
- Justify – make a clear argument for something supported by valid and justifiable evidence

Activity 1.3

Look at the following passages and detect the descriptive, critical and explanation voices. Choose only one for each passage and note down the differences for each.

1. Cystic fibrosis is a condition that is inherited that affects the performance in the lungs and kidneys due to the presence of thick and sticky mucus (NHS, 2016). In the UK, statistics show that one in every 2500 babies are born with the disease. It is suggested that improvements that relate to newborn screening tests have a better clinical condition when compared to patients diagnosed clinically within the first 10 years of life (Dankert-Roelse and Langen, 2011).

2. Cystic fibrosis is a condition that is inherited that affects the performance in the lungs and kidneys due to the presence of thick and sticky mucus (NHS, 2016). In the UK, statistics show that one in every 2500 babies are born with the disease.

3. Cystic fibrosis is a condition that is inherited that affects the performance in the lungs and kidneys due to the presence of thick and sticky mucus (NHS, 2016). In the UK, statistics indicate that one in every 2500 babies are born with the disease. It is suggested that improvements that relate to newborn screening tests have a better clinical condition when compared to patients diagnosed clinically within the first 10 years of life (Dankert-Roelse and Langen, 2011). However, this is not universally agreed due to complications, following screening, leading to a course of treatment when there are no physical signs of respiratory problems (ibid., 2011). The arguments are multifaceted but studies have identified parental factors in screening decisions. One study found parental preference for early diagnosis even if it led to untreatable outcomes (Plass et al., 2010). However, other studies report increased anxiety levels when waiting for additional diagnostic testing (Vernooij-van Langen and Dankert-Roelse, 2011). In summary, parental factors alone cannot sway this argument; further clinical evidence is required and discussed as a major theme of this report.

Answers are at the end of the chapter.

Reports

Often confused with essays and vice versa, reports might contain various different ideas within specific sections. This is the distinction between the traditional essay and a report. Table 1.2 details a typical report structure with supporting explanations of each section.

It is important to check your module guide, as specific guidance will be presented on stylistic measures for assessment. Reports come in all shapes and include different elements. You should always refer to the guidance as set by your HE provider.

Blogs/reflective diary

Throughout your academic and vocational learning journeys, you will be required to reflect on particular tasks that you undertake. These might be assessed through a diary/blog or as part of classroom exercises such as role-playing. Reflection is a key part of your ability to understand your previous and new experiences. Jasper (2003: 2) describes the process of being reflective as 'the way that we learn from an experience in order to understand and

Table 1.2   Report structure

Structure	Explanation
Introduction	● Includes an abstract or executive summary situated at the beginning and provides a descriptive account of the main findings
Main body	● Presents the main ideas and arguments in different sections (these might be numbered)
	● Multiple sections can be used to bring together a variety of ideas that interlink with the main topic, for example:
	1.2 Malaria
	1.2.1. Malaria Prevention
	1.2.2. Malaria Diagnosis
	The above example showcases the topic of Malaria followed by its constituent sections. Each relates to the overarching topic (Malaria) but provides further details on prevention followed by diagnosis
Conclusions	● A comprehensive conclusion drawing upon each section of the report
	● May include a personal reflection section or recommendations
References	● Inclusion of all source types – academic/non-academic
Graphical	● May include diagrams, charts, tables and other graphical illustrations

develop practice'. In this regard, you will learn from an experience before redesigning it for practice based on newly acquired skills. The process is continuous and spirals, as new experiences will arrive and the process is repeated. Documenting this in your studies can be tricky as you are developing skills, knowledge and vocation concurrently throughout a lifelong learning process. Therefore, it is more about taking a snapshot of skill acquisition rather than a description of polished mastery. Fortunately, there are various models and cycles that help you to capture your development – the two you might come across in your programme are Kolb's (1984) Experiential Learning Cycle and Gibbs' Reflective Cycle (1988), which improved Kolb's work in educational reflection theory. Both provide a conceptual framework that you can use in reflective tasks you undertake.

Go Further 1.1

See Chapter 3, Personal and Professional Development, for in-depth detail on how to engage in reflection.

You can find more about Kolb's Experiential Learning as it relates to public health practitioners by following this link to a free article which demonstrates the use of the cycle as an aid to research – 'Reflection as part of continuous professional development for public health professionals: a literature review' – http://jpubhealth.oxfordjournals.org/content/early/2012/10/16/pubmed.fds083.full

See the following link that applies Gibbs' Reflective Cycle to paramedics. It can easily be implemented to a range of health professions and includes some free downloadable content – 'Here's looking at you! An Introduction to Reflective Practice for Paramedics' by Alan Batt (2014) – http://prehospitalresearch.eu/?p=1550

It is not uncommon for students to receive feedback stating the need to be more critical and to bring counter-arguments or differing perspectives into their work. Perhaps the reason behind this is to do with the negative connotations of taking a critical approach. You might think of criticality as the protagonist in provoking or upsetting someone. It is a falsism to criticise personally and act without justification or evidence in any domain, not least academic study. The other factor is to do with learning new material. It is impossible to write critically if we do not have all of the information to hand. This requires an analytical approach because we need to locate, appraise and evaluate material before including it in our work. For example, you might be writing about health and wellbeing – which is a broad area covering many categories, perspectives and actors. Taking the analytical approach requires careful synthesis of all associated parts, identifying crossover relationships and trends when researching material. One way to achieve this is through a concept map. This is a visual method for connecting themes and investigating trends and relationships. Not to be confused with Mind Maps, they are more structured – looking in detail at how (and why in some cases) themes are connected. Figure 1.2 illustrates a basic concept map that investigates health and wellbeing.

The connected arrows indicate the relationship between different parts and the theme. The theme lifestyle has links to exercise, diet and sleep. The visual aspect of creating a concept map helps us to arrange complex information. Our brains are very good at deciphering complex visual material and arranging them into meaningful categories. There are a number of good references online for creating a concept map but the process usually considers the gathering of themes (brainstorming) and organisation – you might use sticky notes to write out themes. Then, a drafting process of laying out material, exploring connections. Finally, these are written to show which themes connect to main and sub-themes. Going through this process enables us to understand important components and their relationship to the topic we are researching. It is a useful starting point for consolidating ideas and preparing for the next step of critical and evaluative writing.

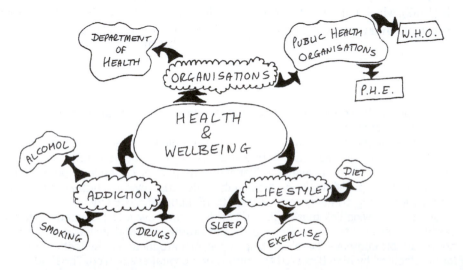

Figure 1.2   Health and wellbeing concept map

After completing a concept map and subsequent investigation into relationships and trends, the next stage will be to write about them, thus moving from the descriptive to the critical and evaluative stages of your assignment. Using the search tips we discussed earlier, you will locate a bank of pertinent scholarly evidence in preparation for writing your assignment. It might be useful to extend your concept map to bridge between the positive and negative arguments about something. A good critical analysis will be balanced and reflective before leading to an overall summation of a topic. In this way, you should remain independent and impartial to what is being said. Your focus is bringing attention to the key arguments and perspectives on said phenomena. Only when a reasoned and justifiable conclusion has been made can it be considered critically approved.

Annotating academic articles

After conducting initial searches, you will have selected one or two academic articles you think are appropriate to your topic. One useful technique to use when narrowing down articles is skim reading. Fortunately, academic articles include an abstract – which is a summary of what the article contains. You will be able to do keyword searches and apply techniques as discussed earlier to highlight anything of importance and focus on the details required.

Think of academic articles as a sales pitch. Recall a time when someone was trying to sell you something. Think about their approach and the language they used. Academic articles won't sell you a car, or anything tangible for that matter, but they will offer you an idea. Authors will use convincing language to grab your attention and get you on their side – so to speak. This isn't a trick or a mind control attempt; instead, articles go through a process of falsification, where other academics review and question the scientific rigor of what is presented and discussed. Personal beliefs will always need support from evidence of studied phenomena. Keep this in mind when developing your own critical concepts.

Thinking critically can springboard you to write critically. Sounds simple, but you need to know what you are looking for. Critical annotation can help so let's start with the following article by Pinsky et al. (2010), who researched the exposure of alcohol advertising to adolescents and young adults in Brazil. Like all good science, the article explains the problem area, introduces us to methods and procedures of how they collected their data, presented results and discussed their findings. Generally speaking, this is how all academic articles are presented. We start to analyse the present article by understanding its main headlines. Let's consider asking the following questions:

- What is the main problem area(s) the article specifically address?
- Who were the participants in the study?
- How did the author(s) go about collecting their data?
- What were the final results and were these positive/negative?

The above will help to shape a descriptive overview, which we include in our final essay. It might be written like this:

Pinsky et al. (2010) researched adolescents and young adults' exposure to alcohol advertising. Through secondary collections and face-to-face interviews, their results suggest that over half (61%) of their sample (N = 1091) [N = the number of people sampled] reported seeing alcohol from different media sources each day (and more than once in each day).

Following the description part, we then move into the critical stage. To help us, let's consider asking the following questions:

- What types of methods did the author(s) use? Were they appropriately performed?
- Was each method viable for each of the results presented? Could there be another way? Provide details on improvements, if any.
- Did the author(s) interpret results accurately through an informed discussion?
- Was there mention of the limitations of the study? What were they? How does this affect the overall results?
- What other evidence is out there to contest/agree with these findings?

The above are some questions that we may ask ourselves when applying criticality. It is useful to make notes in the margin of the paper or use digital markers if preferred. Annotating each section will no doubt throw up further questions, thus it is important to keep the focus on what it was that originally drew your attention to the paper. Always ask yourself – 'how will this article feature in my final assignment?'

Once we have analysed the article we come to add in our critical points. All academic articles will have a limitation section or some reference to how they would either do the study again or some justification on the issues surrounding data collection/analysis. If we run a Control-F search for limitations in our article we locate two mentions (of limitations). Staying with our example, we note the authors mention the 'challenging task to accurately measure media exposure' (Pinsky et al., 2010: 56). This suggests that the term media has multiple uses and may include other types/forms than those asked in the study (e.g., the internet, TV, magazines, etc.). This is rightfully a limitation, as those asked about alcohol exposure might have engaged with another type of media source. Building in our critical element from the descriptive could read like this:

Pinsky et al. (2010) researched adolescents and young adults' exposure to alcohol advertising. Through secondary collections and face-to-face interviews, their results suggest that over half (61%) of the sample (N = 1091) reported seeing alcohol from different media sources each day (and more than once in each day). However, one limitation of the study is the difficulty in contextualising the term media, as participants were prescribed options only in the data gathering stage. In this way, participants might well have engaged with other media sources, such as video games, text messages and music – to name a few. This has implications for the overall inferences and the general difficulty in perusing such research.

The critical element uses information in the article to draw attention to the limitations of this type of research. Indeed, all articles will have their limitations and this enables us to explore critically what exactly is going on. To take this one step further is to review similar studies and compare findings. Here you will build up a better picture of analysis, patterns and trends before offering a well-informed critical appraisal.

INVESTIGATING REFERENCING: STUDENTS' ANATHEMA

Before we start, consider the following syllogism (deductive reasoning in which a conclusion is derived from two premises – Definitions.net, 2016):

I provide references in my work,

References in my work lead to better quality,

Better quality equals better grades, all because I provided references.

To get to its core, referencing deals with the proof and acknowledgement of others' work used in a specific context within your own. When searching for anything, you will select appropriate material to help build an answer against your assignment goals. This takes time, as you will need to search, read and select appropriate literature or other media. Indeed, referencing others' works serves a dual purpose and in its literal sense requires you to show support of a claim by providing a reference from an appropriate source. Consider the following claims and note the differences before selecting the one you think is more trustworthy:

1. Cystic fibrosis has improved over the years mainly due to early diagnosis, targeted therapies, and specialised units.
2. There has been an improvement in the diagnosis, treatment and specialised care for cystic fibrosis patients in recent years (O'Sullivan and Freedman, 2009).

Although written differently, both put out the same idea and seem genuine, both make bold claims about something but only one can be classed as being credible. You should have selected the second claim, as it is supported by an in-text reference. Adding academic references will significantly improve the quality of your work and showcases your knowledge. Again, option two starts this process by including a credible source from a peer-reviewed journal – in this case, *The Lancet*. It will need improving, bringing in alternative views (using and extending upon additional sources) and summarising before moving on. Let's investigate the styles of referencing you will need to master.

Referencing: the basics

Most HE courses will follow the Harvard referencing system to stylise your citations and lists. There are other systems and it is best to read your course handbook or speak to your lecturer should your institution follow a different system. The internet and bookstores are ablaze with guidance on how to develop your referencing skills. One thing to note here is the layout of different media sources (e.g., book, blog, video, audio) that have different reference layouts. This goes beyond this chapter, but there is further guidance in the Go Further link at the end of this chapter.

There are two important steps to remember when using references. Firstly, references that include the author's name, date of publication, title and publisher are located at the back of your work. This is known as your reference list. Secondly, references that are used within your work (known as in-text references or citations) include only the author(s) name(s), the date of publication and a page number if you use a direct quote. These simple rules are the basics of using and applying references into your work. It's a good idea to practise stylistically to get used to different ways to integrate citations into your own work.

In-text references

Let's look at this more closely with examples of how in-text references can be shaped to fit your style of writing and improve its flow. As we have seen previously, writing essays and reports requires various techniques to enable the transition between descriptive, critical and explanatory voices. The following are different in-text styles, the first one suggests a descriptive approach:

- Counihan (2015) suggests that universal peer learning originated in India as a pedagogical package before being shipped worldwide.

The descriptive style might be useful when introducing a new theme or perspective. Alternatively, it can be written with the author's name at the end, but notice the different arrangement with the brackets:

- Universal peer teaching was a pedagogical package that was developed in India before being sent worldwide (Counihan, 2015).

Lastly, we might reference a direct quote. A quotation is used to emphasise a specific point or show support for one of our arguments and it looks like this:

- As Counihan (2015: 291) suggests, 'At the height of its popularity, the method garnered interest from kings, tsars and early educational reformers who were keen to raise standards, particularly access to education for the poor.'

As before, the reference can go at the end of the paragraph or sentence. It depends on the flow of your work and whether the quote is long enough to break away from the main body of text, or short enough to remain as part of the same sentence. There is no universal agreement here so do check course handbooks, but generally, anything longer than three sentences requires indenting and separating from the main body of text. When referencing a direct quote, that is, when you have used exactly the same words as the author(s), you must provide a page number, as can be seen in the brackets above.

Secondary references

As with in-text references, the same process of including a source and placing it near content you have written remains the same, the only difference being the style it is presented in. Sometimes when researching material, we might come across sources we are unable to access, or that information is missing. Let's assume we come across interesting material we found in a book and want to use. However, we cannot gain access to the citation, thus, we think about discarding it. Don't do it! We can still use it by following the basic rules of secondary sourcing.

Let's now look at this in more detail with a worked example. Starting with an extract from an essay we are developing on cystic fibrosis, a secondary reference will be styled like the following:

- In 1959, Gibson and Cooke pioneered a method that revolutionised the diagnosis of cystic fibrosis (cited in Filbrun et al., 2016).

Notice the similarity of providing an author's name and date, the same as we did for our in-text reference in the previous section. However, let's dissect the above into two sentences to master secondary referencing styles.

The first sentence refers to a study completed in 1959 by Gibson and Cooke, and this is what we want to use in our essay. Usually, we would cite it following the *in-text* rules, as before – (Gibson and Cooke, 1959). However, we are unable to find the complete source for our reference list but still want to include it. Therefore, if we consult the second sentence from our example above, we will notice the *(cited in)* reference style. This is because Filbrun and her colleagues *(the et al. part)* have written about the method pioneered by Gibson and Cooke in their own publication. Thus, we are able to acknowledge (and use in our essay/report) the material we want (i.e., Gibson and Cooke) by citing Filbrun and colleagues' book. Finally, you will not need to include the Gibson and Cooke citation in your reference list. Instead, you only include information related to the Filbrun publication. The last Go Further section of this chapter has helpful interactive links and information on how to create a reference list incorporating both in-text and secondary referencing styles.

Referencing will take some time getting used to. Remember to paraphrase sentences into your own words, unless you use a direct quote. Some students consider using multiple quotes to eat up word counts. This won't do, because assessors will want to know what you have understood and whether you can synthesise major arguments, themes and perspectives required at this level of study.

CHAPTER SUMMARY

- You have recognised the transparency in personal skills and how they can be utilised in academic contexts.
- You have investigated, developed and applied techniques for conducting contextualised searches for online material.

- You have understood the assessment processes involved in HE and developed an awareness of descriptive, explanatory and critical voices to be used in academic writing and relative assignments.
- You have taken an in-depth practical look at referencing, its various styles and how it can be applied to academic assignments.

 Answers to Activity 1.3

1. = Explanation
2. = Descriptive
3. = Critical

 FURTHER READING

Websites

These websites will help you with your research skill development:

- The *British Medical Journal* has an excellent resource for reading and researching different types of academic articles and how to read them. It is available at: www.bmj.com/about-bmj/resources-readers/publications/how-read-paper
- See Julian Treasure detail how to give an excellent presentation in his TED talk, which can be found at: www.ted.com/talks/julian_treasure_how_to_speak_so_that_people_want_to_listen?language=en
- Review your referencing skills with *Cite Them Right: The Basics of Referencing*, available at: www.citethemrightonline.com/Basics
- See how to create an end-of-text reference list by viewing this useful YouTube video and channel: www.youtube.com/watch?v=QtfXN8QYJik

Books

These texts will all support your study skills development:

- Burns, T. and Sinfield, S. (2016) *Essential Study Skills: The Complete Guide to Success at University* (4th edn). London: Sage.
- Jasper, M. (2003) *Beginning Reflective Practice*. Cheltenham: Nelson Thornes.
- Kolb, D.A. (1984) *Experiential Learning: Experience as the Source of Learning and Development*. Englewood Cliffs, NJ: Prentice-Hall.
- Lewis, D. (1999) *The Written Assignment: A Guide to the Writing and Presentation of Assignments*. Australia: Kelvin Grove.

REFERENCES

Counihan, C. (2015) Endogenous education in India and the implications of universal peer teaching in the 19th century. In P. Dixon, S. Humble and C. Counihan, *Handbook of International Development and Education*. London: Edward Elgar.

Dankert-Roelse, J.E. and Langen, V.A. (2011) Newborn screening for cystic fibrosis: pros and cons. *Breathe*, 8(2): 4–30.

Filbrun, A.G., Lahiri, T.R. and Ren, C.L. (2016) *Handbook of Cystic Fibrosis*. Switzerland: ADIS Publishing.

Gibbs, G. (1988) *Learning by Doing: A Guide to Teaching and Learning Methods*. Oxford: Oxford Further Education Unit.

Jasper, M. (2003) *Beginning Reflective Practice*. Cheltenham: Nelson Thornes.

Kolb, D.A. (1984) *Experiential Learning: Experience as the Source of Learning and Development*. Englewood Cliffs, NJ: Prentice–Hall.

Lewis, D. (1999) *The Written Assignment: A Guide to the Writing and Presentation of Assignments*. Australia: Kelvin Grove.

NHS (2016) Cystic fibrosis. Available at: www.nhs.uk/Conditions/cystic-fibrosis/Pages/Introduction.aspx (accessed 1 September 2016).

Nightingale, P., Te Wiata, I.T., Toohey, S., Ryan, G., Hughes, C. and Magin, D. (1996) *Assessing Learning in Universities*. Professional Development Centre, University of New South Wales, Australia.

O'Sullivan, P.B. and Freedman, D.S. (2009) Cystic fibrosis. *The Lancet*, 373(9678): 1891–904.

Pinsky I., El Jundi, S.A.R.J., Sanches, M., Zaleski, M.J.B., Laranjeira, R.R. and Caetano, R. (2010) Exposure of adolescents and young adults to alcohol advertising in Brazil. *Journal of Public Affairs*, 10: 50–8.

Plass, A.M., Van El, C.G., Pieters, T., et al. (2010) Neonatal screening for treatable and untreatable disorders: prospective parents' opinions. *Pediatrics*, 125: 99–106.

Sternberg, R.J. (1985) *Beyond IQ: A Triarchic Theory of Intelligence*. Cambridge: Cambridge University Press.

Vernooij-van Langen, A. and Dankert-Roelse, J. (2011) Newborn screening for cystic fibrosis: pros and cons. *Breathe*, 8: 24–30.

2

VALUES AND ETHICAL FRAMEWORKS IN HEALTH AND SOCIAL CARE

Gillian Rowe

Our lives begin to end the day we become silent about things that matter.

Dr Martin Luther King

This chapter will explain the role of values underpinning care in different settings and ask you to evaluate the practical application of the principles of values in care settings. You will also consider your own value base as you understand the theories that sustain ethical practice.

📌 Glossary

- **Anti-oppressive practice** Respects diversity and difference and affirms the autonomy of the people whose health you are working for
- **Code of conduct, code of ethics or code of practice** A guide to the standards of behaviour required in your day-to-day work, and a guide to ethical decision making
- **Confidentiality** Respecting the privacy of information that your patients (clients, service users) give you and ensuring that this information is shared, stored and used in ways governed by the Data Protection Act 1998
- **Courage** Acting in accordance with your personal values, even if this makes you unpopular
- **Delegated duties** Tasks that you perform under the accountability of registered staff
- **Deontology** Ethical rules and laws

- **Empathy** The ability to understand and share the feelings of another
- **Reality ethics** Ethical principles based on virtues
- **Teleology** Seeking good outcomes or consequences
- **Values** A belief in the things we hold to be right and fair
- **Virtues** Characteristics valued as moral goods

INTRODUCTION

What are ethics and values and why do we have them? Philosophers have been pondering the question of how we live and moral responsibility for more than 25 centuries. The earliest written record so far discovered are the codes of Ur, the earliest being the law codes of Urukagina (23 BCE), which attempted to curb corruption by the elite against the poor. The next oldest found code is that of Ur-Nammu (21 BCE), which instituted monetary fines for wrongdoing and the death sentence for murder. The most well known code is that of Hammurabi (17 BCE), which considered notions of justice and fairness, and is the earliest example of the presumption of innocence and the right to a fair trial. The ancient Greek philosophers are divided into those before Socrates (the pre-Socratics) and after Socrates (Socratics). Of the pre-Socratics, Protagoras is the best known, for making the statement 'man is the measure of all things, of the things that are, that they are, and of the things that are not, that they are not' – this means that man decides what is of value and that each person has their viewpoint. Socrates said that 'the unexamined life is not worth living', meaning that we need to be reflective and examine our conscience. This is underscored by Dr Martin Luther King's quote (above), that we need to speak out when we see evidence of wrongdoing.

Science has not always considered the consequences of its actions. Social science experiments have a particularly poor reputation (Stanford prison experiment, Tuskegee syphilis experiment, B.F. Skinner's work with dogs are just some examples). Any research now must go before an ethics committee to ensure the participants are protected and not harmed. The scientists who work with the medical profession have especial ethical considerations, such as that participants in drug trials may be harmed by taking untested drugs or they may be harmed when the drug trial finishes, or that the drug may help them but they cannot have any more until it is licensed.

Recently both the British Medical Association and the Royal College of Nurses voted on whether to support euthanasia. The RCN voted for, the BMA voted against. Everyone gave this their best ethical and moral consideration but arrived at different conclusions.

Working for health is a moral action, for which you need a moral imagination (Kohlberg, 1981); therefore you need to understand your own morals and values, those of your family, your culture and your community, where you, as a person are coming from. You will at times be challenged by competing demands of your physical and emotional resources: trying to do your best when you do not have the equipment or staff you need to do your job properly; trying to put aside your personal feelings when your patient's values challenge your own. Trying to be ethical when you are exhausted requires inner reserves you may not know you possess. This is when you need your moral understanding and ethical framework to support you in your work. Activity 2.1 asks you to think about the values that you have and how you can explore these.

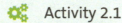

Activity 2.1

Think about the values that you have and how important they are to you, such as not being lied to or having your views respected, and think about how you would feel if they were ignored. You can read more about values in care on the SCIE/Skills for care website (www.scie.org.uk/).

REGULATION OF DELEGATED DUTIES

HCP/HCAs are not currently regulated and therefore work under the supervision of registered nurses. With the creation of the role of Nurse Associate, however, the Nursing and Midwifery Council (NMC) is in the process of setting up a regulatory body that will require registration and its own code of practice. However, codes of practice share many features and so I have included reference to both the NMC code and the Codes of Conduct for Healthcare Support Workers and Adult Social Care Workers in England, Scotland and Wales and used them to highlight how the codes collectively govern your work, especially when engaging in devolved nursing duties. The characteristics of a profession include: using a technical language, accountability, responsibility, autonomy of action, work that is bound by a code of ethics, and a confidential relationship between the practitioner and client and (according to Wickenden, 1952) renders a specialised service based upon advanced specialised knowledge and skill. Healthcare Practitioners (HCPs) and Associate Practitioners (APs) fit these criteria, so the time for your own regulatory body is well overdue.

Until your regulatory body is set up and functioning, accountability rests with the registered staff who supervise your work. They have to ensure that when you are delegated a task:

[1] You have the skills and abilities and are competent to perform it.
[2] That the delegation is appropriate and in the patient's best interests as all patients should expect the same standard of care, whoever delivers it.

Go Further 2.1

The RCN has an advice sheet called 'Accountability and delegation: What you need to know'. It can be found on the RCN website at www2.rcn.org.uk/__data/assets/pdf_file/0003/381720/003942.pdf

Reading this will support your understanding of your role and the role of the person supervising you.

ETHICS IN CARE

We talk about ethics, morals, values and virtues as if the words are interchangeable. *Moralis* is a Latin word meaning morals and is concerned with actions; *ethics* is a Greek word that has a relationship with *ethnos* (ethnicity), and considers what is moral behaviour in any given society. Virtue is about moral excellence (from the Greek *arete* meaning excellence and from the Latin *vir* meaning valour). The Greek philosopher Aristotle considered that if you have good virtues, you can only behave in a virtuous manner. Aristotle also said 'a virtuous action is only moral when it is done with the desire to do the right thing'. The classical virtues are temperance, prudence, justice and courage. Values are principles and standards of behaviour and these can be religious, political or ideological; they are beliefs and attitudes. Putting these principles into action is called a 'social good'. Rawls (1999) discusses the notion of social goods in relation to principles of justice. He considers that each person has an equal right to opportunity and to a share in society's goods.

Ethical philosophy considers how ethical decisions are made and how those decisions are put into practice; they are the why and how we as individuals and as a society work, and each individual society decides its own moral code. There are three main types of ethical enquiry: meta ethics, which examines various societies' attitudes to things; applied ethics, such as the ethical principles used by business or medical ethics; and normative ethics. Normative ethics are the ethics used in healthcare.

Normative ethics

These come in two types: deontology and teleology.

Deontology

Deon comes from *deus*, which means God, so deontological thinking is about duties and rules, such as the Ten Commandments in the Bible. All ethical work takes place within a framework; this might be legal, religious or cultural. Therefore, you need to follow the rules. The main theorist for deontological thinking is Immanuel Kant (1724–1804), who formulated the Categorical Imperative, which is 'Do not act on any principle that cannot apply to all men'. Therefore, when formulating a rule, it must apply to everyone, such as if lying is wrong, then it is wrong for everyone to tell lies for any reason, and you have a moral duty not to lie, even if that results in harm to someone. Deontologists do not consider the consequences of an act. The Categorical Imperative states that moral actions are right or wrong in themselves, without reference to circumstance, therefore truth telling is a moral duty. Kant considered that people should not be treated as 'a means to an end', meaning they should be treated as autonomous individuals and an end in and of themselves.

🗨 Scenario 2.1   Mrs Rivers

Mrs Rivers, aged 74, has just been diagnosed with stage 4 cancer of the bowel; there is evidence of metastasis to the liver. She has refused intervention and wishes to go home to die. She said that she wishes to enjoy what is left of her life but will seek hospice care and pain relief when she needs it. She has asked the nursing staff not to inform her family of her diagnosis as she feels they will pressure her to undertake chemotherapy and surgery. Mrs Rivers' daughter asks you to tell her what is wrong with her mother. She says her mother suffers from depression and is confused at times and is therefore not capable of making her own decisions. What would you do?

Teleology

Telos means 'end' and is the ethics of ultimate purpose; it considers what are the consequential effects of an action. This is broken down into three branches:

- **Act consequentialism**: argues that the morality of any action is dependent upon its consequences. Thus, the most moral action is the one that leads to the best consequences.
- **Rules consequentialism**: argues that focusing only on the consequences of the action in question can lead people to commit outrageous actions when they foresee good outcomes, therefore they say imagine that an action was to become a general rule – if the following of such a rule would result in bad consequences, then it should be avoided even if it would lead to good consequences in this one instance. It is somewhat similar to deontologicalism.
- **Utilitarianism**: devised by Jeremy Bentham (1748–1842) and derives from *utilis* (Latin), meaning useful. Bentham maintained that humans are driven by pleasure and pain, so he devised his hedonist (or felicic) calculus. The calculus determines that an action is right if it produces the greatest good for the greater number of people, and of any two actions, the most ethical one will produce the greater balance over harms. The drawback of the greatest good for the greater number of people is that minorities can be harmed in the process. Read Case Study 2.1 for an understanding of how this works in healthcare.

🗨 Case Study 2.1   Vaccination

Vaccination is a process that can protect the population from preventable contagious diseases; it is a demonstrably successful procedure, however some people refuse to be vaccinated because they feel it is a harmful procedure. If people were forced to be vaccinated, so that 100% of the population were vaccinated, then on statistical probability, some would be harmed. For instance, possibly 1 in every million persons vaccinated for smallpox will die as a result of an adverse reaction but 99.99% of vaccinated people will be protected against the disease. From 1967 to 1980, there was a global eradication pro-gramme to rid the world of this disease (WHO, 2016). There were 4.5 billion (4500 million) people on the planet in 1980 and over 80% of them have been vaccinated; this means a death rate of (very) approximately 4000 adverse reaction deaths. Do you think this was a price worth paying for protection? Would it help to know that from 1900 to 1977, 300 million people globally died from smallpox (WHO, 2016)?

Reality ethics

Bioscience ethicists devised reality ethics to help healthcare workers resolve ethical issues; the principles are based on virtues. Beauchamp and Childress in their classic book *Principles of Biomedical Ethics* (currently in its 7th edition) formulated:

- Autonomy – respect for the individual and their right to choice making.
- Beneficence – do only good and the principle of acting in the best interests.
- Non-maleficence – 'above all, do no harm', stated in the Hippocratic Oath (if you cannot make a situation better, do not make it worse).
- Justice – respect for, and recourse to, the law, which also emphasises fairness and equality.

Added to this is veracity: truth telling and honesty.

CODES OF PRACTICE

Irrespective of whether you work in health or social care, your work is governed by codes of practice: the Nursing and Midwifery Council (NMC) Code of Professional Standards (revised, 2016), which covers health work, the Codes of Conduct for Healthcare Support Workers and Adult Social Care Workers in England, Scotland and Wales and the General Social Care Council Codes of Practice for Social Care Workers and the Northern Ireland Social Care Council Code.

> ### Go Further 2.2
>
> You can download the Code of Practice from the NMC website and the Code of Professional Standards from the Skills for Care website. It is important that you read and understand these as they govern your practice.

What these codes all have in common is a desire to promote ethical practice into your day:

- Respecting people
- Treating people with dignity

- Treating people fairly
- Supporting patients' choices

ANTI-OPPRESSIVE PRACTICE

Before engaging in any intervention, seeking the consent from the patient is critical. Any intervention without consent could be deemed an assault to the individual (read more about consent in Chapter 7, Essential Skills for Care). You need to ensure that the patient has been given enough information to make an informed consent, so that they know what will happen and why. Birkenbach et al. (2012) talks of an 'info-suasive dialogue' as the nature of the informed consent interaction by asking how you can be persuasive without being coercive and thus undermining the patient's autonomy. The medical and nursing profession has a long history of paternalism (we are the experts, and we know what is best for you). There is a knowledge/power differential in healthcare work, but we must acknowledge that the patient is the expert about themselves, therefore the partnership or shared decision-making model is now adopted as the most ethical model when laying out the pros and cons of any intervention. The asymmetrical nature of power and knowledge means that you need to support a patient with decision making, and that the information needs to be presented in a manner that the patients can understand, retain, reflect and decide, then communicate their choice.

Ethical congruence relates to your own understanding of your ethical self, the values that you have and how they are aligned with the values of the organisation for which you work. If you share the same ethical principles, you are more likely to sustain your working relationship.

What the Codes Say 2.1

The NMC Code states that you should (2.1) 'work in partnership with people to make sure you deliver care effectively' and (2.3) 'encourage and empower people to share decisions about their treatment and care' and (2.5) 'respect, support and document a person's right to accept or refuse care and treatment'.

The Codes of Conduct for Healthcare Support Workers and Adult Social Care Workers in England, Scotland and Wales states (2.5): 'always gain valid consent before providing healthcare, care and support. You must also respect a person's right to refuse to receive healthcare, care and support if they are capable of doing so'; and (4.3) 'always explain and discuss the care, support or procedure you intend to carry out with the person and only continue if they give valid consent'.

Some patients may not be able to give informed consent at a time when they need to due to cognitive impairment, or they may lack the capability to give informed consent if their mind is impaired or disturbed. This impairment may be temporary or permanent. Patients need to be assessed using guidance from the Mental Capacity Act 2005. If someone is judged as not having capacity, health workers need to consider what is in the patient's best interests. Family members are usually consulted as they are likely to know the person's wishes if they have not made an advance decision directive (this used to be known as a 'living will'). The main elements to choosing to intervene will be 'can this procedure wait until the patient is able to make their own decision?' and if not, then to try to identify what choices the patients would have made, taking into consideration their personal, religious and cultural beliefs. If no one suitable is available to help, an independent mental capacity advocate (IMCA) must be consulted.

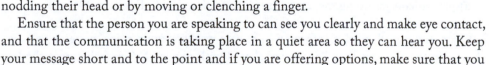

Go Further 2.3

To deepen your knowledge, read about 'Planning for your future' and 'The Mental Capacity Act'on the NHS website.

COMMUNICATING WITH PEOPLE WHO ARE COGNITIVELY IMPAIRED

Communication is the transmission of information, thoughts and feelings (Merriam–Webster online, 2016) but people who are cognitively impaired have difficulty managing this. They may have had a stroke (properly, a cerebral-vascular event), a learning disability, dementia, hearing loss or maybe mentally disturbed, any of which are barriers to communication. Care staff may need to be creative in finding ways to make their message understood; you could try using sign language or Makaton with deaf or LD patients, pictograms, or talk to text systems. Patients may communicate by blinking, nodding their head or by moving or clenching a finger.

Ensure that the person you are speaking to can see you clearly and make eye contact, and that the communication is taking place in a quiet area so they can hear you. Keep your message short and to the point and if you are offering options, make sure that you state them clearly and one at a time.

We have all been in restaurants or cafes where the waiter/ess has reeled off a list of items so fast that you have had to stop them and ask them to repeat what they have said – it's annoying and makes you feel stupid. Sometimes it may be easier for the patient if you ask closed questions which require a yes or no answer, for example, Are you in pain: yes/nod/squeeze finger/blink/groan

It might help to have a family member present who is used to communicating with the patient and can support the conversation, especially if it is regarding consent for treatment, or to help them to understand what the treatment is and how it is going to happen.

RIGHT TO CONFIDENTIALITY

Scenario 2.2   Mrs Rivers (continued)

Mrs Rivers has told you that she does not wish her family to be told of her diagnosis as she feels that they will try to coerce her into accepting treatment. You feel that her family has a right to know and should be consulted, as Mrs Rivers has said she wishes to go home to die and will therefore need their support to do this. Would you encourage Mrs Rivers to tell her family?

The NHS confidentiality policy states that

> All employees working in the NHS are bound by a legal duty of confidence to protect personal information they may come into contact with during the course of their work. This is not just a requirement of their contractual responsibilities but also a requirement within the common-law duty of confidence and the Data Protection Act 1998. It is also a requirement within the NHS Care Record Guarantee, produced to assure patients regarding the use of their information. (NHS England, 2016: 6)

Patients disclose all sorts of information to care workers; quite often, patients will disclose information that they have never shared with anyone before (when was the last time you had a conversation about how often you have a bowel movement?). Care workers expect patients to negate all conversational niceties and give them intimate information. More often than not the patient does, but does so expecting you to fully respect their confidence and not share this information beyond the care setting.

The Codes of Conduct for Healthcare Support Workers and Adult Social Care Workers in England, Scotland and Wales states (5.1) 'treat all information about people who use health and care services and their carers as confidential' and (5.2) 'only discuss or disclose information about people who use health and care services and their carers in accordance with legislation and agreed ways of working'.

Dame Fiona Caldicott's report *A Guide to Confidentiality in Health and Social Care* (2013) was produced for the Health and Social Care Information Centre and it set out five rules regarding the use of confidential information in care settings:

- Rule 1: Confidential information about service users or patients should be treated confidentially or respectfully
- Rule 2: Members of the care team should share information when it is needed for safe and effective care
- Rule 3: Information that is shared for the benefit of the community should be anonymised
- Rule 4: An individual's right to object to their information not to be shared should be respected
- Rule 5: Organisations should put policies, procedures and systems in place to ensure the confidentiality rules are followed

Caldicott considers that 'Confidential information is given on a basis of trust and this is fundamental to safe and effective care'. Sharing information within the care team carries with it the notion of 'implied consent', that the patient has consented for information to be shared with the team in their best interests and for effective care to take place. Care workers need to feel that the care team will also respect their patient's confidentiality and that anyone with access to confidential information is aware of their responsibilities.

Scenario 2.3   Mrs Rivers (continued)

Mrs Rivers has told you that she does not wish her family to be told of her diagnosis. You need to inform your colleagues of her decision so that someone does not inform the family by accident. This information needs to be reported and recorded.

Reporting information to senior staff is crucial to team decision making. Without up-to-date information, mistakes can be made; equally, recording information is critical. Patient notes are legal documents, admissible in a court of law, therefore it is essential that they are accurate records of events. The box below explains how the codes describe this.

> ## What the Codes Say 2.4
>
> The NMC code states (10.1) 'complete all records at the time or as soon as possible after an event, recording if the notes are written sometime after the event', (10.2) 'identify any risks or problems that have arisen and the steps taken to deal with them, so that colleagues who use the records have all the information they need' and (10.3) 'complete all records accurately and without any falsification, taking immediate and appropriate action if you become aware that someone has not kept to these requirements'.
>
> The Codes of Conduct for Healthcare Support Workers and Adult Social Care Workers in England, Scotland and Wales states (4.4) 'maintain clear and accurate records of the healthcare, care and support you provide. Immediately report to a senior member of staff any changes or concerns you have about a person's condition'.

WHY WE RECORD PATIENT CARE

Recording patient care, whatever you do for and with your patient to meet their needs, is essential so the care team know what has taken place. The general rule is that 'if it's not recorded, it didn't happen' and this includes supporting patients with personal care and with nutrition and hydration. Age UK commissioned a report called *Hungry to Be Heard* in 2006 and its follow up, called *Still Hungry to Be Heard*, in 2010. The original report found that older patients were either admitted to hospital malnourished and nothing was done about it, or became malnourished in hospital because they didn't get the right food or the help needed to eat it. The RCN carried out a survey of nursing staff to explore attitudes towards nutritional care. While 81% of nurses thought nutrition was 'extremely important', 42% felt there was not enough time to devote to patients' nutrition. They listed barriers as: not enough staff to help patients eat or to monitor intake, conflicting priorities, and poor choice and quality of food (RCN, 2007). The exercise was repeated in 2010, and found that while improvements had been made, they were inconsistent and some people were still lacking nutritional support. For people with learning difficulties the situation was far worse. The report *Death by Indifference* (Mencap, 2007, 2012) revealed 74 deaths due to malnutrition or dehydration and Mencap alleges NHS institutional discrimination against people with learning difficulties. In 2014, 95 patients died of starvation or dehydration on a hospital ward and 15 died in care homes from the same cause; the figure was higher in 2015 (Office of National Statistics, 2017). It has been reported that ward doctors are prescribing water, to ensure patients are given drinks. Many Trusts are making improvements and some Trusts are training band 4 staff as link nurses to ensure nutrition is supported and recorded. Nutritional support is now a key line of enquiry within the CQC inspection process.

Go Further 2.4

Read the *Hungry to be Heard* and *Death by Indifference* reports. They are challenging to read as they are evidence of poor care and neglect; however, they will help you to become a better care worker.

📺 Scenario 2.4   Mrs Rivers (continued)

Mrs Rivers has a poor appetite. The Trust runs a 'red tray' scheme and has protected mealtimes. It has been noticed that Mrs Rivers is losing weight, but staff mark this down to her disease progression (cachexia) and she has not been proposed as a 'red tray' patient. You notice that when the catering staff bring the next meal trolley, they ask her if she is hungry and when she says 'no' they pass on to the next bed. When you check Mrs Rivers' notes, no food intake has been recorded since her admission. Do you think this is because she hasn't eaten or that it hasn't been recorded? Without accurate records, how can you be sure, and think about how this sits with non-maleficence and safeguarding principles?

WHAT ARE THE 6 Cs?

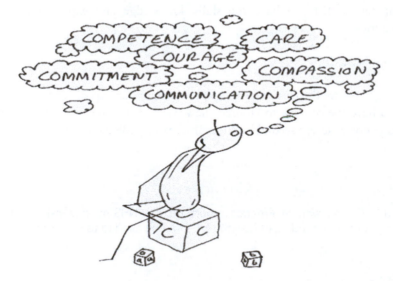

Figure 2.1   The 6 Cs

The changing nature of ethics in healthcare has moved from obligation (deontology) to responsibility (consequentialism). An early exponent, Tronto (1993), said 'there is a pre-existing moral relationship between people; therefore, the question is, "How can I meet my caring responsibility?"' The dreadful events at Mid Staffordshire NHS Foundation

Trust led some to believe that modern nurses suffered from moral blindness and were able to 'pass by on the other side' as they were not moved to alleviate their patients' suffering and accept their caring responsibility. The subsequent report by Robert Francis QC (Francis, 2013) made 290 recommendations, and the NMC acted against several nurses who were struck off the register. One of the recommendations by Francis was to examine the way that student nurses are educated and to introduce value-based training. This initiated the '6 Cs' of care to underpin *Compassion in Practice* by Bennett and Cummings (2012).

- Care: 'Care is our business' means that we work at individual, family and population level. It means prevention, early intervention and health promotion as well as treatment of ill health.
- Compassion: means that we give care using sympathy, empathy, respect and dignity, which has been described as 'intelligent kindness'.
- Communication: this relates to communication skills with your patients, with your colleagues, with team members and the wider caring community. It also considers the communication you have with your patients and is central to 'No decisions without me'.
- Commitment: a commitment to care for your patients in the best way that you can.
- Competence: that you have the skills, knowledge and expertise to carry out your duties.

Last but not least

- Courage: to have the personal strength to speak out and speak up for your patients, and to have the courage to embrace new ways of working for your patients. The courage not to accept second best for either your patients or for yourself.

Go Further 2.5

Read the *Compassion in Practice* report on the NHS nursing vision website to deepen your understanding of how the 6 Cs can be applied to your practice.

CONTINUOUS PROFESSIONAL DEVELOPMENT

 ### Scenario 2.5   Mrs Rivers (continued)

Mrs Rivers still hasn't told her family about her diagnosis. You are concerned that her daughter has said she suffers from depression; this isn't in her nursing notes but you are aware that she is refusing food. You wonder if she would benefit from some grief counselling but you do not have this training or skill. What is the most beneficial thing that you can do for this patient?

Knowing when you don't have a skill for an activity is important. If you can identify gaps in your training, you can then find the means to gain skills by asking your mentor to find a training provider, if one is not available within the workplace.

> ## What the Codes Say 2.5
>
> The NMC code states (22.3) 'keep your knowledge and skills up to date, taking part in appropriate and regular learning and professional development activities that aim to maintain and develop your competence and improve your performance'.
>   The Codes of Conduct for Healthcare Support Workers and Adult Social Care Workers in England, Scotland and Wales states (1.6) 'Strive to improve the quality of healthcare, care and support through continuing professional development'.

TRUTH TELLING

The almost seventh C is that of candour, the duty to tell the truth and speak out. The RCN guidance states 'Generally, the law imposes a duty of care on a healthcare practitioner in situations where it is "reasonably foreseeable" that the practitioner might cause harm to patients through their actions or omissions'. The NMC and GMC (2015) have produced a guidance on the Duty of Candour called *Openness and Honesty when Things go Wrong: The Professional Duty of Candour*. Alasdair MacIntyre (2007) discusses truth telling from a virtue perspective, considering honesty, courage and justice are virtues in practice.

Scenario 2.6   Mrs Rivers (continued)

Mrs Rivers is deeply upset; she tells you that someone has shared her diagnosis with her son. As she suspected, he wants her to have treatment, he is coming back this evening with his sister to have a family meeting to decide their way forward. Mrs Rivers said her wishes have not been respected and her confidentiality breached. She says she wants to discharge herself and go home as she no longer trusts the hospital staff.

Ethical contradictions

Mrs Rivers feels her rights have clearly been disregarded, she is distressed as this is a conversation she wished to avoid for as long as possible. The staff member who disclosed her diagnosis did not respect her autonomy. Autonomy is the individual's right to make decisions on their own behalf, whereas non-maleficence is the healthcare worker's duty to do no harm. However, the staff member may consider that as the son asked for his mother's diagnosis, s/he felt s/he could not lie to him on deontological principles and that he had a right to know, and the principles of beneficence and non-maleficence have a place in evaluating truth telling and non-disclosure. The staff member who made the disclosure might argue that s/he acted for 'the greater good'; that the deontological principle of confidentiality should be overridden by teleological principles. It has been argued that respecting the autonomy of the individual does not imply a one-size-fits-all approach to truth telling. There may also be cultural considerations; in many cultures the family is informed before the patient, as they are considered as having primary decision-making responsibility.

What the Codes Say 2.6

The NMC code states (4.1) 'balance the need to act in the best interests of people at all times with the requirement to respect a person's right to accept or refuse treatment', (5.5) 'share with people, their families and their carers, as far as the law allows, the information they want or need to know about their health, care and ongoing treatment sensitively and in a way they can understand' and (16.4) 'acknowledge and act on all concerns raised to you, investigating, escalating or dealing with those concerns where it is appropriate for you to do so', also (17.1) 'take all reasonable steps to protect people who are vulnerable or at risk from harm, neglect or abuse'.

The Codes of Conduct for Healthcare Support Workers and Adult Social Care Workers in England, Scotland and Wales states (1.1) 'Be accountable by making sure you can answer for your actions or omissions'.

The codes have some contradictions. On the one hand, you need to respect the patient's autonomy on the right to accept or refuse treatment; on the other hand you need to act in the best interests of all and share information, and you must be accountable for your actions or omissions. Mrs Rivers might argue that she is vulnerable to pressure from her family and is therefore at risk of abuse. She feels her daughter will ask to have her mental capacity assessed. If Mrs Rivers is found to lack capacity, do you think this would mitigate the breach of confidentiality?

Privacy is the right of individuals to keep information about themselves from being disclosed. Patients are in control of information about themselves. Patients should decide with whom, when and where to share their health information. Therefore, a disciplinary offence has taken place. The responsibility to maintain confidentiality is defended by the principle of beneficence, which asserts that health workers should act in ways that prevent harm and promote good to others. NHS Trusts' legal responsibility is explicitly stated in the Confidentiality Policy (DH, 2003): 'Patients, staff, members and the general public have a right to expect that NHS Trusts are a confidential environment in which their information will be treated with due care and respect, shared only with their consent, in their best interests or through a legislative duty'. All Trusts and care providers will have their own version of the Confidentiality Policy and it is your responsibility to read and understand them.

Whistleblowing

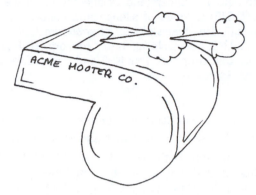

Figure 2.2   Whistleblowing

Activity 2.2

You were on duty the day the breach was committed and you have a good idea who made the disclosure. You feel that action should be taken against the staff member, but it seems to have been 'brushed under the carpet', and your manager seems deaf to your comments. How would you deal with this?

The Public Disclosure Act 1998 supports staff who 'whistleblow' on poor practice. In the past, employees were reluctant to raise concerns about wrongdoing because they feared that they would not be listened to or that they would be putting their jobs at risk. The Act allows employees to voice authentic concerns about misconduct and malpractice without receiving penalties such as dismissal, victimisation, or denial of promotion, facilities or training opportunities. Certain types of disclosures qualify for protection if they are made in good faith, and if the disclosure tends to show that the misconduct is happening now, happened in the past or will likely happen in the future. The staff member who made the disclosure probably did so believing they were acting in the family's best interests and who probably would, under the same set of circumstances, do the same thing again. Before taking any complaints out of the organisation, you need to discuss your concerns with your manager to give them the opportunity to address them. However, the 'deaf effect' (Mannion and Davis, 2015), which occurs when 'the decision-maker does not hear, ignores or overrules a report of bad news' (Cuellar, 2007), can lead to frustration and hostility by the whistleblower, who may then pursue an external course of action.

Go Further 2.6

Read this article to help you understand whistleblowing in the NHS: Mannion, R. and Davies, H. T. (2015) Cultures of silence and cultures of voice: the role of whistleblowing in healthcare organisations. *International Journal of Health Policy and Management*, 4(8): 503–5. Available at: http://doi.org/10.15171/ijhpm.2015.120. Also, read 'The Public Disclosure Act from NHS and Social Care perspectives' which is available on the NHS website.

All employers should have a 'whistleblowers' procedure which must be adhered to if you are to be protected. Please be warned that undertaking whistleblowing is not for the faint-hearted. Although you are protected by law, sometimes the law is not enough and whistleblowing has affected careers and obstructed job opportunities; it is an act of courage to speak out. Francis (2015) stated 'When an NHS worker speaks up, they are making a vital contribution to the quality and safety of patient care. This is true not just for doctors, nurses, and other qualified healthcare professionals, but of all NHS workers regardless of position.'

Go Further 2.7

You can read the executive summary of the Francis Report online: www.gov.uk/government/publications/report-of-the-mid-staffordshire-nhs-foundation-trust-public-inquiry

---

Ethical decision making

In order to make ethical decisions, you need some tools, the best known being David Seedhouse's ethical grid. It is a four-layer diagrammatic grid containing ethical connections that need to be considered. In the centre is the person (autonomy), layer 2 considers the virtues of truth telling, beneficence (do only good) and non-maleficence (do no harm). Layer 3 could be considered teleological, as it considers what is good for the person, the family and society, and layer 4 could be considered deontological as it considers laws, codes and risks. Seedhouse (2008) states

> The Ethical Grid is a tool, and nothing more than that. Like a hammer or screwdriver used competently, it can make certain tasks easier, but it cannot direct the tasks, nor can it help decide which tasks are the most important. The Grid can enhance deliberation, it can throw light into unseen corners and can suggest new avenues of thought, but it is not a substitute for personal judgement. (2008: 209)

The grid can provide some coherence when mulling over the best way forward through a moral maze. Seedhouse also considers where any agent stands in terms of ownership of the decision-making process, using his 'rings of uncertainty'. For a full explanation of using the grid and rings, read David Seedhouse's book, *Ethics: The Heart of Healthcare* (see Further reading).

CHAPTER SUMMARY

- You have been introduced to the study of ethics in healthcare, to understand that there is more than one way of determining the right moral action.
- Deontology considers what are the rules, what does the law say you should do; teleology asks what are you trying to achieve, and how you can secure the best outcomes for patients and their families.
- Reality ethics considers the application of virtuous practice: doing only good, not making things worse, acting fairly and being honest. I have included excerpts from the various codes of practice; these give you a framework to work within, to guide your work and to give you support when you are challenged to justify your practice.
- You have looked at the tools you might use to make sure you have considered all the stakeholders when making an ethical decision that affects patients, their families and the wider community. Remember that your work must take place within these frameworks in order to be ethical.

FURTHER READING

All these codes, articles and books are mentioned in the text and will help you to deepen your understanding of ethics in your working practice. The codes are regularly updated and freely available on the internet.

Codes

- The NMC Code of Practice
- The Codes of Conduct for Healthcare Support Workers and Adult Social Care Workers in England, Scotland and Wales
- The British Association of Social Workers Code of Ethics
- HCPC Standards of Conduct, Performance and Ethics

Report

- Francis, R. (2013) *The Mid Staffordshire NHS Foundation Trust Public Inquiry* (Chaired by Robert Francis QC). Report of the Mid Staffordshire NHS Foundation Trust. London: HSMO.

Books

- Armstrong, A. (2010) *Nursing Ethics: A Virtue-Based Approach*. Basingstoke: Palgrave.
- Banks, S. (2012) *Ethics and Values in Social Work* (Practical Social Work Series). London: Palgrave/BASW.

- Melia, K. (2013) *Ethics for Nursing and Healthcare Practice.* London: Sage.
- Seedhouse, D. (1998, 2008) *Ethics: The Heart of Health Care.* Chichester: John Wiley.

Journal article

- Mannion, R. and Davies, H.T. (2015) Cultures of silence and cultures of voice: the role of whistleblowing in healthcare organisations. *International Journal of Health Policy and Management*, 4(8): 503–5.

REFERENCES

Age UK (2006) *Hungry to be Heard: The Scandal of Malnourished Older People in Hospital.* London: Age UK. Available at: www.ageuk.org.uk/documents/en-gb/hungry_to_be_heard_inf.pdf?dtrk=true (accessed 10 April 2017).

Age UK (2010) *Still Hungry to be Heard: The Scandal of People in Later Life becoming Malnourished in Hospital.* London: Age UK. Available at: www.ageuk.org.uk/documents/en-gb/for-professionals/health-and-wellbeing/id9489_still_hungry_to_be_heard_report_28ppa4.pdf?dtrk=true (accessed 10 April 2017).

Beauchamp, T. and Childress, J.F. (2013) *Principles of Biomedical Ethics*, 7th edn. Oxford: Oxford University Press.

Bennett, V. and Cummings, J. (2012) *Compassion in Practice: Nursing, Midwifery and Care Staff. Our Vision and Strategy.* London: DH and NHS Commissioning Board. Available at: www.england.nhs.uk/wp-content/uploads/2012/12/compassion-in-practice.pdf (accessed 10 April 2017).

Birkenbach, A., Singer, H. and Litan, R. (2012) An empirical analysis of aftermarket transactions by hospitals. *Journal of Contemporary Health Law & Policy*, 28(1): 23–38.

Caldicott, F. (2013) *A Guide to Confidentiality in Health and Social Care: Treating Confidentiality with Respect.* Leeds: Health & Social Care Information Centre. Available at: http://content.digital.nhs.uk/media/12822/Guide-to-confidentiality-in-health-and-social-care/pdf/HSCIC-guide-to-confidentiality.pdf (accessed 18 May 2017).

Cuellar, J. (2007) Security and trust management. *Computer Science*, Vol 6710. Berlin: Springer.

Department of Health (2003) *Confidentiality: NHS Code of Practice.* London: DH. Available at: www.gov.uk/government/uploads/system/uploads/attachment_data/file/200146/Confidentiality_-_NHS_Code_of_Practice.pdf (accessed 10 April 2017).

Francis, R. (2013) *The Mid Staffordshire NHS Foundation Trust Public Inquiry* (Chaired by Robert Francis QC). Report of the Mid Staffordshire NHS Foundation Trust. London: HSMO.

Francis, R. (2015) *Freedom to Speak Up: An Independent Review into Creating an Open and Honest Reporting Culture in the NHS.* Available at: http://freedomtospeakup.org.uk/wp-content/uploads/2014/07/F2SU_web.pdf (accessed 10 April 2017).

Kohlberg, L. (1981) *The Philosophy of Moral Development.* New York: Harper and Row.

MacIntyre, A. (2007) *After Virtue: A Study in Moral Theory*, 3rd edn. Indiana: University of Notre Dame Press. First edition published in 1981.

Mannion, R. and Davies, H.T. (2015) Cultures of silence and cultures of voice: the role of whistleblowing in healthcare organisations. *International Journal of Health Policy and Management*, 4(8): 503–5.

Mencap (2007) *Death by Indifference: Following up the* Treat Me Right! *Report.* Available at: www.mencap.org.uk/sites/default/files/2016-06/DBIreport.pdf (accessed 10 April 2017).

Mencap (2012) *Death by Indifference: 74 Deaths and Counting. A Progress Report 5 Years On.* London: Mencap. Available at: www.mencap.org.uk/sites/default/files/2016-08/Death%20by%20Indifference%20-%2074%20deaths%20and%20counting.pdf (accessed 10 April 2017).

Merriam–Webster online (2016) *Communication.* Available at: www.merriam-webster.com/dictionary/communication (accessed 19 June 2017).

NHS England (2016) *Confidentiality Policy.* Leeds: NHS England. Available at: www.england.nhs.uk/wp-content/uploads/2016/12/confidentiality-policy-v3-1.pdf (accessed 10 April 2017).

Nursing and Midwifery Council and General Medical Council (2015) *Openness and Honesty when Things go Wrong: The Professional Duty of Candour.* Available at: www.nmc.org.uk/globalassets/sitedocuments/nmc-publications/openness-and-honesty-professional-duty-of-candour.pdf (accessed 8 June 2017).

Office for National Statistics (2017) *Deaths from Dehydration and Malnutrition, by Place of Death, England and Wales, 2014 to 2015.* Available at: www.ons.gov.uk/peoplepopulationandcommunity/birthsdeathsandmarriages/deaths/adhocs/006520deathsfromdehydrationandmalnutritionbyplaceofdeathenglandandwales2014to2015 (accessed 20 June 2017).

Rawls, J. (1999) *A Theory of Justice.* Harvard, MA: Harvard University Press.

Royal College of Nursing (2007) *Nutrition Now. Principles for Nutrition and Hydration.* London: RCN.

Seedhouse, D. (2008) *Ethics: The Heart of Health Care.* Chichester : John Wiley.

Tronto, J. (1993) *Moral Boundaries: A Political Argument for an Ethic of Care.* London: Routledge.

Wickenden, W. (1952) Professional organisations and professional schools. *Journal of Engineering Education.*

World Health Organization (2016) *Smallpox.* Available at: www.who.int/csr/disease/smallpox/en/ (accessed 10 April 2017).

3
PERSONAL AND PROFESSIONAL DEVELOPMENT

Gillian Rowe

Personal development begins with self-awareness. You get to know who you really are; your values, beliefs and the dreams you wish to pursue. True fulfilment can never come from chasing other people's dreams.

Abraham Maslow (1954)

This chapter is aimed at helping you become an independent learner and will help you to become an effective student. It will also support you to become a reflective learner and develop the skill of reflective writing and journal keeping. It will also introduce you to evidence-based practice and team working.

 Glossary

- **Personal development** Improves your self-identity and self-awareness
- **Professional development** Earning or maintaining your professional credibility
- **Reflection** Giving serious thought or consideration to something
- **Reflective guide** Using a guide to help you clarify your thinking
- **IT** Information Technology

INTRODUCTION

Personal and professional development is a lifelong process, and as Abraham Maslow so nicely puts it, it begins with self-awareness, getting to know who you are and what your strengths and challenges are. The world of health and social care changes rapidly; new ideas, changing legislation, improving standards and different ways of working all add to the changing landscape. Continuous development comes about by reading journals, taking courses and attending seminars or conferences and deepening your understanding of how change affects what you do and how you do it. A good example of this is in Chapter 2 on values and ethical frameworks, which discusses the changes brought about by the Francis Report and the introduction of the 6 Cs into your day-to-day work.

Becoming a student and adopting an enquiry-based outlook is a big change in your life; it is hard work and demands that you put aside time to engage in study. It also asks that you question what you do and how you do it, and this learning process is formularised by using reflective practices such as journal keeping. This chapter will guide you through the process and sits alongside Chapter 1 on academic study skills, which will support you in your academic work.

GETTING STARTED

Independent learning requires commitment and discipline. To make it easier for yourself, try to organise a study space. The family dining table doesn't really cut it as you will need to move your stuff continually (and things will get lost). You will need somewhere to put all the books you buy and borrow, and your folders. This could be a big box (at least it is all together), a filing cabinet and desk, or your own study room. Your study space needs to be free of distractions, so keep clutter to a minimum.

You will need a personal computer or laptop and an internet connection, and a software package such as MS Student, as you will need a range of office software (e.g., Word, PowerPoint, Publisher and Excel in MS Office). Apple Mac for students requires an institutional log in but they also offer deals. Linux offer their office suite equivalent free but there may be compatibility issues.

Being IT literate

If you are not computer literate, you will struggle to create work to an acceptable standard. You might consider approaching your local college or training provider to enrol on an IT course. You will need to use basic office packages and they will support you with this. Some of these courses are free so ask around before paying for training. Check with your local JobCentre as they might sponsor you if you are unemployed.

Learning resources

Books are another big budget item. You will need various key texts for each module you study, and although there will be a few copies of each book on the reading list in your college library, usually they are restricted to 7- or 14-day loans. Buying your books secondhand from a previous student or by checking out deals on eBay or Amazon is a good way to get reasonably priced text books.

Your college may well subscribe to an ejournal account such as Athens, which will allow you free access to health journal articles; however, these subscriptions are remarkably expensive and smaller colleges without university partnerships may not afford them. In which case, most journal publishers have 'open access' articles which are free to view. Colleges may also have institutional subscriptions to relevant monthly publications (such as *Nursing Times*) which should be in the library. Always remember that the librarian is your friend and will help you obtain books and articles through the college book exchange system.

BECOMING A STUDENT

When you are a beginning student, it is easy to feel intimidated by how much you must learn – it seems endless. There is a new language to learn, long complicated words that you need to spell, understand and use. You may feel that you do not bring anything to the table in the classroom, or that your views are not of value. However, everyone has knowledge and experience of value and you will develop confidence as you read and learn more and this will help you find your voice. Do not feel scared to put your hand up and ask if you do not understand something; you will not be the only one and you will probably be doing your shyer classmates a favour. Remember that you can watch YouTube channels such as Khan Academy or Bosman Science, and also read your module textbooks to support your learning. Textbook publishers often have online learning materials too to support the textbook content.

You can join online forums dedicated to the knowledge you seek, watch TED talks and take free online courses such as edX or futurelearn. All the information you need is available but ensure you use reputable sites (there is a lot of misinformation, fake news and downright rubbish out there too).

LEARNING ABOUT HOW YOU LEARN

To complete a higher education degree or higher apprenticeship you need to think about how you learn. Everyone has a learning style; you may well have completed an assessment of your learning style when you were younger, but our learning styles change as we get older.

Think about the differences in the way you learnt at school or FE college (where you may have done A-Levels, BTEC or NVQs). Look at Table 3.1 to see how you will learn on university-level programmes.

Table 3.1   Types of learning

Learning at lower level	Learning at higher level
Information given by teachers	Self-directed learning
Listening	Active participation
Shared responsibility for learning	Personal responsibility for learning

In order to take responsibility for your own learning, you need to understand how you learn. Google the Honey and Mumford (1982) learning style assessment and find out what kind of a learner you are; this will help you to tailor your learning to suit your style. You may be familiar with VARK, which means Visual, Audio, Reading and Kinetic. Most people have more than one preferred way of learning so compare your VARK style with your Honey and Mumford assessment: activist, pragmatist, reflector and theorist. Use Table 3.2 to tick all the words that apply to you.

Table 3.2 Learning styles: Tick the words that apply to you

Activist	☐	Reading	☐
Pragmatist	☐	Kinetic	☐
Reflector	☐	Logical	☐
Theorist	☐	Social	☐
Visual	☐	Solitary	☐
Audio	☐	Verbal	☐

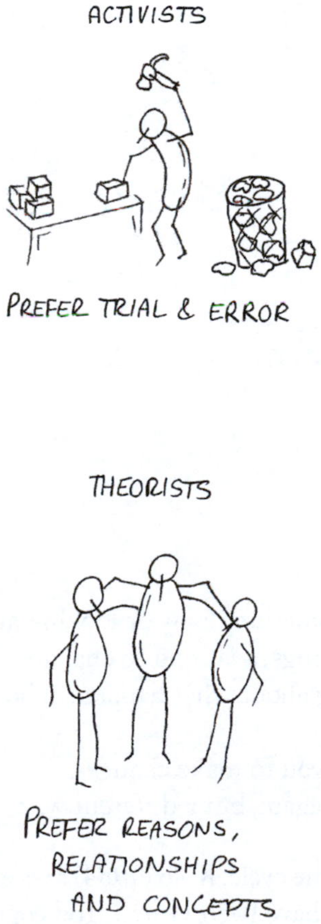

Figure 3.1 Learning styles

There are other learning styles, but they mainly extend or add to this list.

So what is learning? The online Oxford Dictionary (2016) says it is 'the acquisition of knowledge or skills through study, experience, or being taught'. Learning always involves change in your disposition, your thinking and your capability. It is also concerned with the acquisition of knowledge that can be applied and retained. Learning is said to take place when you can make sense of something and reinterpret it into your own words and can apply something into a skill or action. Kong Qui (better known as Confucius) was a Chinese philosopher in the 4th century BCE and he said 'By three methods we may learn wisdom: first, by reflection, which is the noblest; second by imitation, which is the easiest; and third by experience, which is the bitterest' (www.britannica.com/biography/Confucius, 2016). Experience can be gained from poor decision making which is then used to make good decisions (bitter experience), but David Kolb (1984) designed the Experiential Learning Cycle as a way of learning and practising.

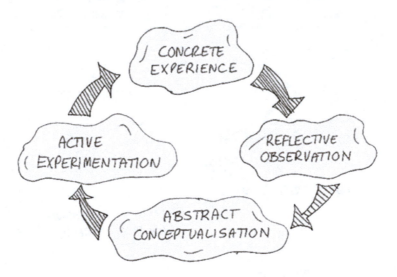

Figure 3.2   Kolb's Experiential Learning Cycle

[1] Concrete experience might be trying something new or looking at a known thing in a new light, or a new way of doing things, adapting to change.
[2] Reflective observation is about thinking about what happened, how you did, what went well, what didn't work.
[3] Abstract conceptualisation can prompt you to make changes.
[4] Active experimentation means doing it again, but a different way.

And this takes you back to the beginning of the cycle. Kolb (1984) says effective learning takes place when all four parts of the cycle have been visited. The cognitive psychologist Jean Piaget (1964) said that children learn through a process of assimilation and accommodation, that they build on knowledge (called scaffolding). They start out with a schema (an idea) which may be used in different situations (assimilation) or changed (accommodation) when the schema doesn't work. He considers that equilibration drives children's search for understanding, and balance comes from mastery. Piaget only applies his theory to children, not adult learners, and focuses on development not just learning, but you can see a relationship between this model and the Kolb model.

Generally, the students most likely to succeed are students who attend lectures. There is a direct correlation between attendance and achievement. It is not always the brightest student who achieves the highest degree classification but the one who has a willing attitude and an enquiring mind. By adopting what the psychologist Carol Dweck (2006) calls 'a growth mindset', which is a belief that talent will only get you so far, whereas hard work and dedication makes for great accomplishment. No one achieves great things without years of effort and practice. Once you know how you learn, you can consider the barriers to your learning. Table 3.3 is based on a survey I conducted with students to identify their barriers. Do any of these apply to you?

Table 3.3   Thinking about the things that can get in the way of your studies

I'm terrible at time management – always have been!	☐
I know what I need to do – I just can't make myself do it	☐
I can't work unless I'm under pressure	☐
I'm just lazy – no other explanation!	☐
I always leave everything to the last minute – it's just the way I am!	☐
I never have enough time to do what I want	☐

GOOD TIME MANAGEMENT

We have all been here, even your lecturers! However, unless you really are the kind of person who is able to sit up all night and hand in a first-class paper, it will help if you can plan your time management for the next 15 or 30 weeks of study. Go Further 3.1 explains that poor time management can result in students leaving their course.

Go Further 3.1

Students often report that their inability to manage their time is the biggest problem they face when trying to fit in everything that has to happen in the home, at work and study. A study by Goldfinch and Hughes (2007) cited Yorke (1999) who found that a 'lack of self-management skills and/or study skills is commonly given as a reason by younger students for withdrawing from their degree programme'. On their website, the National Union of Students (NUS) have an advice page to help you with time management.

Non-study obligations

Keeping a weekly record is critical to staying on track. Some weeks will be the same but others may need to accommodate trips to medical facilities either for yourself or another family member, children's sports day, parents evening, creating a birthday party or going to a wedding (try not to arrange your own wedding in term time) and learning to drive. Do not forget to programme in household chores such as shopping, cooking, washing and cleaning.

Moving house or finding a new home is something that happens a lot for students. It is better to move in the term breaks if possible. Moving is stressful enough without the added burden of study, and universities generally do not accept moving (other than in emergency) as a reason for an extension on your hand-in dates.

Organising childcare and planning how to cope when it falls apart, or when the children are sick, is important. You might have a job and work regular hours or shifts and these needs should be programmed in. You might also work irregular hours or night shifts or be on call; somehow these must be accommodated. Students are noted for having a hectic social life and therefore you should be no different and this needs to be considered when planning your study time. Also, try to give yourself some 'me' time to unwind. Look at Activity 3.1 and consider if this activity would help you with time management.

 Activity 3.1   Make a time planner

Google 'printable weekly planner' and download and print some copies off, filling them in at the beginning of each week. This activity will add evidence for your portfolio as well as keeping you up to date on your studying.

If you are keeping a weekly diary, use backward planning. When you write a due date in your diary/planner, go back a week and give yourself a reminder that the due date is approaching.

It really is essential that you keep track of 'hand-in dates'. Here sticky notes are your friend.

Use a colour-coding system. Keep some coloured sticky notes on hand and use those for reminders that a due date or other important events is approaching. For instance, use a yellow (amber) sticker to serve as a warning seven days before your assignment is due in, and a red one for two days before hand in.

Think about the things that soak up your time, called time sponges. Look at Table 3.4 and see how many you waste time on.

What can you do?

Deactivate Facebook or use it as reward for two hours spent studying. Do Activity 3.2 to decide what would work for you.

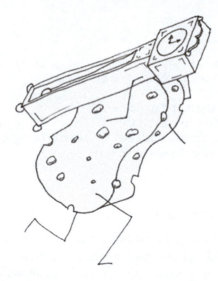

Figure 3.3   Time sponge

Table 3.4   Time sponges: How many of these do you waste time on?

Friends' Facebook pages	☐
Checking your overdraft	☐
Snapchatting your overdraft page capture	☐
Checking out boohoo/Molly Louise/Amazon/eBay	☐
Twitter	☐
Pinterest	☐
Facebook (again ...)	☐
Making a cup of tea	☐
Instagramming a picture of your cup of tea	☐
Television/iPlayer/YouTube/Pokémon	☐
Opening a new tab ... Facebook again	☐

⚙ Activity 3.2   Make a chart of your time sponges

Your personal time sponges	What may work for you

(Continued)

(Continued)

When we perceive tasks as difficult, inconvenient, or scary, we may shift into pro-crastination mode with self-sabotaging statements.

- I'll wait until I'm in the mood to do it.
- There's plenty of time to get it done.
- I work better under pressure so I don't need to do it right now.
- I've got too many other things to do first.

Getting started and staying on track

- Complete small tasks straight away rather than putting them off. This will encourage you to begin tackling larger tasks needing attention.
- Break difficult or 'boring' work into sections. This allows you to approach a large task as a series of manageable parts.
- Don't try to write a whole assignment in one sitting. Write it section by section.
- If you have 'writer's block', try writing something – anything – down. Even if you change it completely later, at least you have made a start. The alternative is having nothing at all.
- Make a Mind Map of your assignment title. This should give you the main key words.

If you find yourself losing direction, sit back and think of why you are doing this course, remembering your goals can put everything into perspective.

Summary of key stages in managing your time

- Organising your study time – give yourself treats and rewards, take frequent short breaks away from your books or computer. Run around the block or to the park and back to get your circulation flowing.
- Planning ahead – be organised and aware of both work and social commitments.
- Prioritisation – discover what needs to be done by when, expect to study at home for at least two hours for each hour spent in class.
- Action planning – how will you complete tasks and stay motivated?
- Evaluating your progress on a regular basis – how are you getting on and are you on schedule?

UNDERTAKING A SWOT ASSESSMENT

SWOT is an acronym for Strengths, Weaknesses, Opportunities and Threats. You can identify things in each area that either support your learning or are barriers to your learning. Use Table 3.5 for some ideas to help you to write this. Once you have identified your barriers (weakness and threats) consider how you might overcome them and what changes you may need to make.

Table 3.5   Ideas for a SWOT assessment

Some ideas for Strengths or Weaknesses	Some ideas for Opportunities or Threats
Time management Work ethic Confidence Communication skills Empathy Ability to follow instructions Showing initiative Can work in a team Independent Understand confidentiality Tactful Patient Reliable IT literate Flexible Numeracy skills Relevant work experience Social skills Working under pressure Organised Multi-tasking	Available time for study Student finance Job availability Pay/salary Family Current employment Government policies Skill set Travel time Educational support/study support Relationships

BECOMING REFLECTIVE

> Research has shown that the regular habit of journal writing can deepen students' thinking about their course subjects by helping them see that an academic field is an arena for wonder, inquiry, and controversy rather than simply a new body of information. (John Bean, 2001)

What is reflection, and why do we do it? Reflection is something of an art and a skill; it is the process of mulling over our day and thinking about events that may have puzzled us. The purpose of reflection is to facilitate learning from experience and develop critical thinking; it can also enhance your problem-solving skills. Engaging in higher education and higher vocational training teaches you to learn to think as effectively as you learn to write. Academic life gives you the opportunity to reflect on your college learning, such as a thought-provoking lecture or tutorial or reflecting on the feedback of your submissions which might give you advice on how to improve your work.

You must learn to have an open mind, to not be judgmental, and to examine your thought processes. Your reflective journal is more than a simple account of your working day – it is an examination of your working day. As Bean (2001) (quote above) so rightly says, reflection can allow you to experience the wonder of your learning, being totally amazed or shocked by new knowledge. A part of the reflective process is the willingness to self-criticise, to change or challenge beliefs, actions, assumptions and practice. Trevithick (2000) suggested 'The use of self-knowledge or self-awareness in professional practice involves the conscious employment of social work skills, knowledge, values and personal experience in ways that are illuminating to the work in hand', therefore you are encouraged to develop courage and independence in thinking.

Professor Jenny Moon (2006: 162) says that 'we reflect on things that are relatively complicated. We do not reflect on a simple addition sum – or the route to the corner shop. We reflect on things for which there is not an obvious or immediate solution'. John Dewey (1933) said, 'Reflection has two interconnected qualities, that of being troubled by some phenomenon and doubting the evidence, and of searching for answers which will remove the problem and doubt.' Reflection is about self-learning and seeking answers; it is also about being self-aware as it involves your beliefs, values, qualities, strengths and limitations. When engaging in reflection you are considering your role, actions and inactions in any given situation. Do Activity 3.3 and see how engaging in reflection supports your learning about your practice.

Activity 3.3

Think about an event that has occurred, something that made you stop and think. Reflection is a conscious action and gives you the opportunity to evaluate the experience. Learning journals are not usually written in 'the third person', you can say 'I think' or 'I feel' and this gives you an authentic voice in your work.

What happened? (Describe)	What was my role in this? (Analyse)
How did I feel about this? (Evaluate)	What did I learn? (Self-awareness)

Reflective guides

We often use a reflective guide to aid reflection. This is because sometimes it is hard to look at something from other perspectives or take on board other people's views. By using a guide, we can examine an experience from 360 degrees. The most commonly used guide is Gibbs Reflective Cycle (1988), but all reflective cycles have similar components (see Figure 3.4).

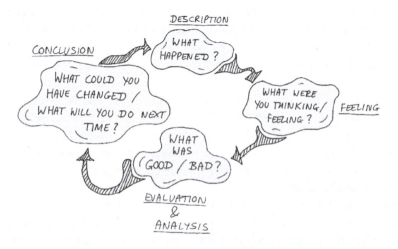

Figure 3.4 Reflective cycle

Table 3.6 Schön's two types of reflection

Reflection on action	Reflection in action
Reviewing that occurs after an event	Continually assessing while actually acting

Donald Schön (1984) wrote extensively on the value of reflection (mainly in education) but his work considered two types of reflection: reflection on action and reflection in action (Table 3.6).

Schön considers the ability to reflect in action as 'professional artistry'; this means that if a situation develops while participating in an activity, you are able to intervene, respond and make changes. He states

> The practitioner allows himself [*sic*] to experience surprise, puzzlement, or confusion in a situation which he finds uncertain or unique. He reflects on the phenomenon before him, and on the prior understandings which have been implicit in his behaviour. He carries out an experiment which serves to generate both a new understanding of the phenomenon and a change in the situation. (1984: 68)

Quite often in healthcare we are presented with an 'accepted picture', which may be based on preconceived ideas, received wisdom or unconscious bias; we become reflective when presented with information that does not fit this accepted pattern and engage in 'retrospective' reflection. To become reflexive thinkers and engage in conscious processing, we need to attend to our intuitive thoughts (Rolfe, 2001). Read Scenario 3.1, and think about how reflection has helped Anya to support her client.

Scenario 3.1   Mr Smith

Mr Smith suffers from dementia and lives in a dementia care unit. His behaviour at meal times is puzzling. He happily eats breakfast and supper, but will not eat his lunch. At lunch time he pushes his chair back, leaves the table and sits in an armchair. Anya (the senior care worker) found that if she brought him a biscuit and a cup of tea, he would accept these. At a team meeting Anya discussed his behaviour with her manager and she asked if she could organise a family meeting to find out how to resolve this situation and support his nutritional needs.

Anya met with Mrs Smith, who told Anya about Mr Smith's life. She said he was a proud man, who had worked as a miner in the coal industry. They worked hard to buy a house and raise their children, and there was little spare money. Mr Smith insisted that they saved up if they wanted something new as he was afraid of getting into debt. They had had family holidays, usually staying in 'Bed and Breakfast' guest houses near the coast.

After Mrs Smith had left, Anya wondered about where Mr Smith thought he was now; she knew from conversations she had with him that he was not orientated to time and location but he knew he was not at home. Anya mulled over Mrs Smith's comment about Mr Smith being a proud man and his attitude to money. The next day at lunch time, when Mr Smith was assisted to the table, he again pushed his chair away. Anya said to him that lunch had already been paid for but Mr Smith still went to the armchair. Anya rang Mrs Smith and related the

(Continued)

(Continued)

day's events. Mrs Smith said that Mr Smith usually paid cash when they were out for lunch. The following day, when Anya was supporting Mr Smith with getting dressed, she put some money in his pocket and told him it was to pay for his lunch. At lunch time, she assisted him to the table and reminded him to pay for his food with the money in his pocket. Mr Smith put the money on the table and ate his lunch.

● Apply the Gibbs cycle to this case study. How many times did Anya go through the cycle?

By applying reflective practice, Anya was able to support Mr Smith with his nutrition in a way that he was comfortable with.

Some journal work will be based on your clinical experiences; these will be structured around the patient's care. Your structure might be (1) Objective (or goal) of an intervention, (2) Outcome (good, neutral, poor), (3) Evaluation (did the intervention work), (4) Plan (amend the care plan). Each of these headings will require links to theoretical models of care and reflective thinking.

Keeping a reflective journal

Those of you who have completed NVQs will be familiar with the concept of 'naturally occurring evidence'; this is learning that takes place as you go about your day-to-day work. Keeping a reflective journal is a way to capture this evidence and gives you an opportunity to see how your knowledge and skill grow over time.

A reflective journal is different from a personal diary, as it examines your professional practice; it also does not need daily recording but should be used regularly. Your placement mentor may ask to see your journal, so ensure that you respect confidentiality and do not identify patients/clients/staff or settings by name or places.

Which format you use for your journal is up to you – it could be a paper portfolio, an e-journal or a personal blog or vlog, or you might need to use your training organisation's e-portfolio system. Either way, it must be kept securely and password protected.

It is also a way of keeping things in perspective when you are feeling overwhelmed in placement. Sometimes traumatic things occur which you need to make sense of, or you have experienced a difficult or challenging situation, or maybe you have worked in a team that has achieved success (good things need to be thought about too).

Your journal is also a good place to make links between theory and practice as well as making notes on research you have undertaken (or need to undertake) to support your learning. By keeping a journal in clinical practice, you have something to look back on to support your report or essay writing or your observed structured clinical examination (OSCEs).

Journal work must be honest. Try to faithfully capture the experience so that you can analyse and evaluate the situation; you need to question your actions and consider if you would do the same thing again in the same situation or if you would change your action and consider how this would affect an outcome. It might be useful to write your experience down and revisit it a few days later when you have had time to assimilate events or calm down if something has upset you. Your views might change or you may have deepened your learning by research or talking to your mentor.

How should a journal be written?

Each entry of the journal will have its own agenda and requirements. As you develop your skill in reflection, Moon (2008) says you should move from basic description to profound evaluation. Therefore, you should travel along a continuum:

Reflective aspects > Critically reflective aspects > Analytical and evaluative aspects

(Adapted from Hatton and Smith, 1995)

Table 3.7 shows you the different reasons for keeping a journal.

Table 3.7   Reasons to keep a journal

Reflect on doing something for the first time
Challenge received wisdom
Think about how this experience connects with previous experiences
Record key events and experiences
Clarify or provide solutions to problematical issues
Provide a means to extend knowledge and skills
A place to experiment with and develop writing styles
Increase your self-awareness
Evaluate your personal and professional growth
Store ideas or material that could be used in an assignment

Your learning journal

When you write your journal, you are engaging in independent learning, and you are writing about things that are meaningful to you. It is an opportunity to make links with disparate information from different sources such as class notes, handouts, conversations you have with your mentor/patients/clients/ward staff. Your writing can also identify gaps in your knowledge and guide your research.

Evidence-based practice

Your journal can also contribute to your knowledge of evidence-based practice (EBP). This practice marries together the principles of clinical expertise, best-evidence research and the patients' values and feedback. The integration of these things can help support the patient care process, develop and understand your practice, why decisions are made, lessons you have learnt and implication of these for your future practice. David Sackett

(1996) said that evidence-based practice is 'the conscientious, explicit and judicious use of current best evidence in making decisions about the care of the individual patient. This means integrating clinical expertise with the best available clinical evidence from systematic research.' Adopting the principles of EBP into your thinking and reflection shows that you are willing to learn from experience and to change things, and that you are open to new ideas and new ways of supporting your patients.

You will want to consider:

- What internal/external factors were influencing you?
- What knowledge/values did or should have informed you?
- How did your actions match your beliefs and knowledge?
- What factors made you act in incongruent ways?
- What are you going to do the same or differently in this type of situation next time it happens?

Read the article recommended in Go Further 3.2 to gain a better understanding of EBP.

Go Further 3.2

Read *Critical Thinking and Writing for Nursing Students* by Bob Price and Anne Harrington (2016) which is freely available under 'Example essays' at: https://uk.sagepub.com/en-gb/eur/critical-thinking-and-writing-for-nursing-students/book245638#preview. The authors discuss a reflective piece written by 'Raymet' who speculates on her patient 'Mrs Drew' and how to manage her pain control. It is also a good example of how to write a reflective essay.

TEAM WORKING

Healthcare practitioners will always be part of a team, whether you are in a care setting, clinic, domiciliary working or on a ward, therefore team working skills are essential. Teams come together for different purposes and small teams will be part of a larger grouping. Look at Table 3.8 to get an idea of who is in a multi-disciplinary team (MDT) and a multi-agency team (MAT). Multi-disciplinary teams consist of the staff within a setting, while multi-agency teams are part of the wider health and social care community.

The King's Fund states that

> Where multi-professional teams work together, patient satisfaction is higher, healthcare delivery is more effective, there are higher levels of innovation in ways of caring for patients, lower levels of stress, absenteeism and turnover, and more consistent communication with patients. (The King's Fund, 2017)

Teams that work well are clear in their roles and goals and support each other in achieving them; effective teams therefore experience less stress. The value of multi-disciplinary

Table 3.8   Multi-disciplinary teams and multi-agency teams

Multi-disciplinary teams	Multi-agency teams
Matrons/Nurses (RGNs/RMNs/Midwives)	Health visitors
Healthcare Assistants	Community matrons/nurses (RGNs/RMNs/Midwives)
Healthcare Practitioners/Nursing Associates	Domiciliary sport workers
Doctors/Surgeons/Anaesthetists/Consultants	Social workers
Therapists	Police/Probation officers/Youth Offender Teams
Diagnosticians	Youth workers
Dietitians	Therapists
Paramedics	Housing support workers

teams is that alternative and competing perspectives are carefully discussed leading to better quality patient care. Teams who meet regularly with a clear shared purpose, and are a mix of the organisation's hierarchy and are seated in the premise of person-centred care, can provide effective service to the patient.

Working in a team

While you are at college, you will probably experience working in a team. The team members may have chosen themselves or you may be allocated a team. Good teams, however, don't just happen; you need a common purpose and everyone needs to contribute using their skills, talents and knowledge.

Tuckman (1965) first described the mechanisms involved in creating teams and named them 'Forming, Storming, Norming, and Performing' (Figure 3.5). The first role of the team is to appoint a leader or organiser who has the responsibility of ensuring

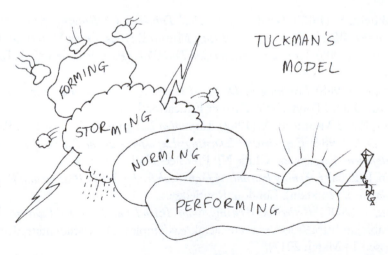

Figure 3.5   Tuckman's model

the team achieves its objectives. The forming stage involves the team getting to know each other and becoming familiar with the goals; this can be an anxious time and the team leader needs to take a dominant role to get the ball rolling. Quite often the team has meetings about setting realistic and achievable objectives and will use such aids as a Gantt chart or Prince2 so that the objectives are planned and agreed in a timely manner.

The storming stage is the trickiest, as this is when the purpose of the goals and the leadership role are challenged. Quite often conflict arises as people have different ways of working or disagree with approaches to problem solving. Members may withhold their cooperation or leave the team at this stage. If the team survives this then they move on to norming, which is when the team accepts their role, starts to socialise together and works collegially. It then achieves the performing stage and works effectively without friction and the leader can step back or delegate part of the role as the team functions well.

CHAPTER SUMMARY

- You have been introduced to the skills of being a successful student, including preparing to study, learning how to study and learning how to identify your barriers to study.
- You have also learned how to become reflective and keep a reflective journal.
- It has introduced you to notions of evidence-based practice and given you some theoretical underpinning of team working for health and social care both at placement and in college.

FURTHER READING

Reading these texts will deepen your understanding of study skills and reflection:

- Brookfield, S. (1987) *Developing Critical Thinkers: Challenging Adults to Explore Alternative Ways of Thinking and Acting*. Milton Keynes: Open University Press.
- Dweck, C. (2006) *Mindset: How You Can Fulfil Your Potential*. New York: Ballantine Books.
- Gibbs, G. (1988) *Learning by Doing: A Guide to Teaching and Learning Methods*. Oxford: Oxford Polytechnic, Further Education Unit.
- Honey, P. and Mumford, A. (1982) *Manual of Learning Styles*. London: Palgrave.
- Kolb, D.A. (1984) *Experiential Learning: Experience as the Source of Learning and Development*. Englewood Cliffs, NJ: Prentice–Hall.
- Moon, J. (2006) *Learning Journals: A Handbook for Reflective Practice and Professional Development* (2nd edn). London: Routledge.
- Moon, J. (2008) *Reflective Writing: Some Initial Guidance for Students* [online]. Available at: http://services.exeter.ac.uk/cas/employability/students/reflective.htm (accessed 14 March 2017).

- Price, B. and Harrington, A. (2016) *Critical Thinking and Writing for Nursing Students* (3rd edn). London: Sage.
- Schön, D. (1984) *The Reflective Practitioner: How Professionals Think in Action*. New York: Basic Books.
- Thompson, S. and Thompson, N. (2008) *The Critically Reflective Practitioner*. Basingstoke: Palgrave Macmillan.

REFERENCES

Bean, J.C. (2001) *Engaging Ideas: The Professor's Guide to Integrating Writing, Critical Thinking, and Active Learning in the Classroom*. San Francisco: Jossey–Bass.

Dewey, J. (1933) *How We Think*. Boston: Heath and Co.

Dweck, C. (2006) *Mindset: How You Can Fulfil Your Potential*. New York: Ballantine Books.

Gibbs, G. (1988) *Learning by Doing: A Guide to Teaching and Learning Methods*. Oxford: Further Education Unit, Oxford Polytechnic.

Goldfinch, J. and Hughes, M. (2007) Learning styles and success of first-year undergraduates. *Sage Journal Active Learning in Higher Education*, 8(3): 259–73.

Hatton, N. and Smith, D. (1995) Reflection in teacher education: towards definition and implementation. *Teaching and Teacher Education*, 11(1): 33–49.

Honey, P. and Mumford, A. (1982) *Manual of Learning Styles*. London: Palgrave.

Kolb, D.A. (1984) *Experiential Learning: Experience as the Source of Learning and Development*. Englewood Cliffs, NJ: Prentice–Hall.

Maslow, A. (1954) *Motivation and Personality*. New York: Harper.

Moon, J. (2006) *Learning Journals: A Handbook for Reflective Practice and Professional Development* (2nd edn). London. Routledge.

Moon, J. (2008) *Reflective Writing – Some Initial Guidance for Students* [online]. Available at: http://services.exeter.ac.uk/cas/employability/students/reflective.htm (accessed 13 March 2017).

Oxford Dictionary (2016) *Learning*. Available at: https://en.oxforddictionaries.com/definition/learning (accessed 19 June 2017).

Piaget, J. (1964) *The Psychology of the Child*. New York: Basic.

Rolfe, G. (2001) *Critical Reflection for Nursing and the Helping Professions: A User's Guide*. Basingstoke: Palgrave Macmillan.

Sackett, D. (1996) Evidence based medicine: what it is and what it isn't. *BMJ*, 312.

Schön, D. (1984) *The Reflective Practitioner: How Professionals Think in Action*. New York: Basic Books.

The King's Fund (2017) *Improving NHS Culture: Teamworking*. Available at: www.kingsfund.org.uk/projects/culture/effective-team-working (accessed 17 March 2017).

Trevithick, P. (2000) *Social Work Skills: A Practice Handbook*. Maidenhead: Open University Press.

Tuckman, B. (1965) Developmental sequence in small groups. *Psychological Bulletin*, 63: 384–99.

4

LEADERSHIP AND TEAMWORK IN HEALTH AND SOCIAL CARE

Michelle Henderson

The NHS needs people to think of themselves as leaders not because they are personally exceptional, senior or inspirational to others, but because they can see what needs doing and can work with others to do it.

Turnbull-James (2011: 18)

This chapter will develop your awareness of the background to leadership and management in the current care sector contexts. As you work through the chapter, you will understand key leadership skills and qualities and how the use of reflection contributes to your professional development, and how you should seek leadership opportunities irrespective of your grade or position within your workplace.

Glossary

- **Care Quality Commission (CQC)** The regulatory and inspection body for health and social care
- **Emotional intelligence** Defined as self-awareness, self-regulation and a level of empathy and understanding of others' perspectives
- **Healthwatch** Healthwatch England established as an effective, independent consumer champion for health and social care
- **Leadership** Having vision and the skills to implement change
- **Management** Managing people, resources and budgets
- **The Berwick Review (2013)** This report is about patient safety, which includes the importance of leadership

- **The Francis Report (2013)** The findings following investigation into the failings at Mid Staffordshire NHS Trust
- **The Shape of Caring Review (Raising the Bar) (2015)** This document looks at the overarching value of high quality education for the caring professions with a focus on HCAs and nurse associate roles

INTRODUCTION

It is never too early to start thinking about leadership in healthcare regardless of the stage you are at in your healthcare career. Leadership has never been more important. Changes to the way healthcare is commissioned, increasing use of technology and the financial challenges faced require those working in health-care to utilise skills of leadership regardless of position or grade. Across boundary working between statutory, private and voluntary providers and the changing land-scape of how services are delivered means leadership skills are crucial. Change is constant but quality remains paramount. On the back of the Francis (2013), Keogh (2013) and Berwick (2013) reports, leadership skills are seen as central to achieving this.

We all need to start thinking about leadership at all levels of healthcare. It is therefore recognised that those embarking on careers in healthcare and study-ing professional programmes need to understand the importance of leadership in current contexts

Leadership can no longer be seen as positional-related, exclusive to those at the top or at certain stages of their careers or training – leadership skills are required at all levels. Literature supports a move away from traditional hierarchical approaches (The King's Fund, 2011); leadership is about working with, and inspiring others. Leadership skills are required when you are mentoring, involved in project work or carrying out your day-to-day duties, and therefore it is important to start to think about your views of leadership, and how you can develop leadership skills within your role and beyond. The aim of this chapter is to introduce you to leadership within healthcare practice and to enable you to start thinking about the concept and skills development you will need early in your learning journey. The first part of the chapter will look at what is leadership, examining the current debates between leadership and management. The second section will look at why leadership is important and how it impacts on quality of care. The final section will explore skills for leadership development, including the value of self-assessment and reflection, looking after your own wellbeing and identifying learning opportunities.

LEADERSHIP VS. MANAGEMENT – WHAT'S THE DIFFERENCE?

There are many debates about the differences between leadership and management.

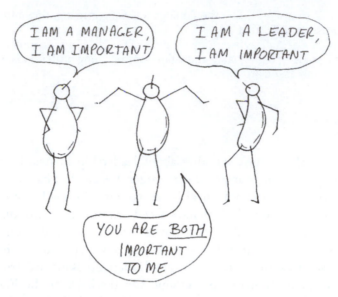

Figure 4.1   Leaders and managers are both important

John Kotter provides a definition:

> Management is a set of processes that keep an organisation functioning. They make it work today – they make it hit this quarter's numbers. The processes are about planning, budgeting, staffing, clarifying jobs, measuring performance, and problem-solving when results did not go to plan. Leadership is very different. It is about aligning people to the vision that means buy-in and communication, motivation and inspiration. (Kotter, 1996: 25)

However, the difference is not as clear-cut as Kotter's definition written almost 20 years ago. Ellis and Abbott (2014) argue they are interchangeable and that, indeed, all good managers are likely to also be good leaders. In a financially challenging climate, it could be argued that this is essential in order to utilise and maximise resources. A report in the *Health Service Journal* argues we focus too much on definitions, and identifies that we should look more towards action for practice to reduce bureaucracy to maximise leadership resources in the NHS (HSJ, 2015).

Whilst leadership may be seen as the skills to sell vision, or motivate individuals towards a vision, how this is achieved may be dependent on someone's leadership style or how they utilise power (which will be covered later on in this chapter). Therefore, to suggest that all leaders are capable of selling a vision and motivating others may be inaccurate, as not all leaders achieve such goals, in fact some fail spectacularly. We therefore may need to start to think about the title we give to people as leaders and what is actually meant by leadership and management. This might not always mean those traditionally seen as being in charge or at the top.

Whilst some literature may argue the differences between leadership and management and attempt to make them distinct in their roles, it is key to remember that both have a valued role within healthcare. Management ensures the day-to-day workings run smoothly, managing resources, people and budgets for example. Without these sets of skills many key functions in healthcare would not occur. If we think of leadership as setting direction and inspiring vision, it is clear to see how such skills are important to ensure change is moved forward.

It is important to remember that managers can be leaders and leaders can be managers, or these can be very separate individual roles. Instead of comparing leadership vs. management, it is therefore suggested that perhaps such roles should be seen as a circle; a continuum of interaction dependent on circumstance and situation, neither one more important than the other, and how leadership skills should be developed by all involved in healthcare regardless of formal job tittle.

Figure 4.2 highlights some of the differences and similarities of leadership and management.

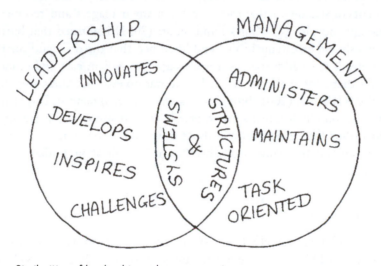

Figure 4.2 Similarities of leadership and management

💬 Scenario 4.1   Ali

Ali is a lead clinical educator who wants to implement a new training package with staff in a large theatre department of over 80 staff. He has great vision of how it will be put in place and it would lead to a formal qualification. Why might the lead clinical educator need to work with the theatre manager (who has overall day-to-day responsibility for the department) to put this training in place?

Go Further 4.1

Read the full NHS Leadership Review:

Rose, S. (2015) *Better Leadership for Tomorrow*. NHS Leadership Review [online]. Available at: www.gov.uk/government/uploads/system/uploads/attachment_data/file/445738/Lord_Rose_NHS_Report_acc.pdf

WHERE ARE WE NOW? A SNAPSHOT OF MANAGEMENT AND LEADERSHIP

> If Florence Nightingale was carrying her lamp through the corridors of the NHS today, she would almost certainly be searching for the people in charge.
>
> (The Griffiths Report, 1983)

Over 30 years ago, the Griffiths report (1983) looked at management within the NHS. The report author Sir Roy Griffiths made this statement as he was concerned at the lack of management in the NHS. The report remarked on the absence of management or leaders who held responsibility and attempted to encourage a role for clinicians more closely involved in management decisions and created the vision of the general manager. Fast forward to 2011, and The King's Fund (an independent charity) still identifies that those in clinical roles need to be engaged more in managerial decisions. There have been comments or statements that there are 'too many managers' and 'too many chiefs and not enough Indians'. The King's Fund report (2011) identified that both leaders and managers should be of equal value and identified that the disregard for the value of managers needs to be addressed as it is damaging to patient care and morale of the workforce. Furthermore, the report argued there was no evidence there were too many managers. The NHS Plan (2001) brought back the (modern) matron. This came off the back of a public consultation that showed people wanted strong visible leadership. The plan also identified that leadership was about drive and innovation, not just seniority, and a move towards all those involved in healthcare thinking about leadership, and their role within this.

Mid Staffordshire failings

In 2008, Mid Staffordshire NHS Trust was investigated due to its high mortality rate. What was uncovered identified one of the most significant failings the NHS has seen since its inception. Key factors identified from the initial investigations were the lack of management and leadership. In 2010, a full public enquiry was launched, chaired by Sir Robert Francis QC. The final report identified reasons why things went so wrong and the report made many recommendations. The main themes suggested a need to encourage a culture of openness and transparency; a system of accountability for all; a system promoting clinical leadership that put patients first as a priority in achieving this.

Following on from the Francis Inquiry, in 2013 Sir Bruce Keogh was asked to lead a review of 14 hospital trusts which had persistently high mortality rates. Eleven of the 14 trusts inspected were put into special measures and scheduled for re-inspection, and the review report set out key areas for improvement of care. Again, the importance of leadership and management featured within this report. Professor Berwick was asked to look at how 'zero harm' could be made a reality in the NHS. The Berwick Review (2013) made in total ten recommendations with core themes around transparency, continual learning, regulation and seeking patient and carer opinions. At the heart of all the themes that emerged was the need for leadership, and those willing to promote high standards and speak up when things are going wrong.

Since the enquiries following the Mid Staffordshire failings, there has been many published documents attempting to address the key issues of ensuring that such failings do not occur again and that developing leadership skills can help to achieve this goal.

Go Further 4.2

To find out more about this, read the full report:

Francis, R. (2013) *Report of the Mid Staffordshire NHS Foundation Trust Public Inquiry: Executive Summary*. London: TSO.

⚙ Activity 4.1

The King's Fund, an independent charity, has undertaken much research into leadership in healthcare. Read the following documents commissioned by The King's Fund:

- The King's Fund (2014a) *Culture and Leadership in the NHS*. Available at: www.kingsfund.org.uk/publications/culture-and-leadership-nhs
- The King's Fund (2014b) *Developing Collective Leadership for Health Care*. Available at: www.kingsfund.org.uk/sites/files/kf/field/field_publication_file/developing-collective-leadership-kingsfund-may14.pdf
- The King's Fund (2015) *The Practice of System Leadership: Being Comfortable With Chaos*. Available at: www.kingsfund.org.uk/publications/practice-system-leadership

What are the themes throughout the three publications on the position and view of leadership in healthcare today?

How does this fit with your experiences of practice? Consider writing a short reflection on the differing aspects of leadership.

Frameworks for leadership

The *Five Year Forward View* (NHS England, 2014) talks about strong leadership and supports the value of the NHS Leadership Academy – a national organisation responsible for leadership training and development in the NHS. The review by Lord Rose (2015), *Better Leadership for Tomorrow*, recognised that change was full scale in the NHS, but perhaps people in the frontline of services were not fully skilled or prepared to participate in this change. It emphasised the importance of seeking out talent and developing staff, and considered the importance of equipping them with the right skills and direction to meet the challenges.

Working across boundaries and organisations is an example of such current challenges. West et al. (2015) argue there is urgent need for leadership across boundaries within and across organisations. This means working collectively and cooperatively, which is in effect collective leadership. Financial challenges and the way the NHS is changing in terms of how it delivers services, is requiring those working in it to have different sets of skills as services can no longer run in isolation. West et al. (2015) consider that collective leadership is more crucial due to the changing nature of service provision. Czabanowska et al. (2014) state that a horizontal approach to leadership and working with others rather than a top-down approach is required, meaning leadership skills and behaviours that foster inclusion, collaboration and engagement in sharing leadership roles regardless of position or grade should be encouraged.

The *Shape of Caring Review (Raising the Bar)*, published by Health Education England in March 2015, focused on the role of the care assistant and the development of the Associate Practitioner role, firmly putting value on unqualified roles within healthcare and their importance to frontline care. Establishing such roles also requires a focus on leadership development in staff who may not previously have had any formal leadership development opportunities.

Leading Change, Adding Value (NHS England, 2016) is a national framework that recognises the value nurses have in leadership, and strongly promotes leadership to achieve the 'triple aims of: better patient outcomes, better patient experiences and better use of resources'. It suggests that as the face of healthcare changes, healthcare workers will need to have coaching and mentoring skills, be able to support patients and work with others, and be confident practitioners which will in turn require leadership skills.

A new national framework that acknowledges the importance of leadership development demonstrates the current value and drive that is being placed on leadership into 2017 and beyond. NHS Improvement (2016) launched *Developing People – Improving Care*, a multi-agency effort. It aims to address four key themes:

- Developing systems leadership skills
- Improvement skills for staff at all levels
- Compassionate, inclusive leadership skills
- Talent management, developing people and investing in leaders of the future

Go Further 4.3

Deepen your knowledge and understanding of current practice by reading:

NHS Improvement (2016) *Developing People – Improving Care: A National Framework for Action on Improvement and Leadership Development in NHS-funded Services* [online]. Available at: https://improvement.nhs.uk/uploads/documents/Developing_People-Improving_Care-010216.pdf

So what does all this mean for those embarking on a career in healthcare? Current demands on the health service require those working in it to be aware that change is constant, that those working in it should have an understanding of the importance currently being placed on leadership skills, and that we need to stop thinking of leadership as being someone else's role. Utilising and developing confidence in leadership skills can have benefits for patient care, and for personal and professional development.

WHY IS LEADERSHIP ESSENTIAL FOR TEAM WORKING?

> Teamwork is essential in the provision of healthcare. The division of labour among medical, nursing and allied health practitioners means that no single professional can deliver a complete episode of healthcare. (Leggat, 2007: 11)

Evidence is clear where teams work well staff feel more engaged and deliver better care. Leadership is central to this and the development of leadership skills is the starting point to contributing to a positive team working culture. Collaboration is required in a healthcare system that now crosses boundaries between statutory, non-statutory and voluntary services.

The importance of human factors such as how teams work together, is crucial in terms of impact on patient safety (WHO, 2009). Teams bring together a range of skills both technical and personable, bring diversity and different perspectives. Learning to work with others is essential. Part of the journey is beginning with understanding how your own leaderships skills can influence your position in team working. NHS England (2014) identifies that the five-year forward view sets a vision for work across community and hospitals and removing the barriers between the two areas traditionally worked in silo. Ham (2014) recognises within teams, the influence of respected team members can be as powerful as those with positional power and therefore we can all contribute and play a valuable role within team working.

Case Study: Dorothy

Dorothy is brought to the A&E in an ambulance after being found collapsed at home by her neighbour. The initial impression by the clinical team is Dorothy looks like she may have had a stroke

- Which members of the MDT (multi-disciplinary team) will have inputted into Dorothy's care so far from the moment her neighbour dialled 999?

Dorothy is moved to a medical ward for further care. She is starting to improve but her neighbour confides to a nurse that she has been struggling for a while and finds it difficult to climb the stairs. Dorothy's only son lives in Australia. Medically, Dorothy is well enough to build towards going home but still has some weakness from her stroke. .

- Which members of the MDT may be involved at this stage?

Assessment finds Dorothy is not safe to return to her own home alone, a social worker will now liaise with social services and care providers to get Dorothy back to her own home with support.

- As the named person looking after Dorothy so far, why is it important to be working with all the MDT members to build towards discharging her home?
- What skills may you need to manage all the different assessments and updates occurring in Dorothy's care between the MDT members involved?

LEADERSHIP AND QUALITY OF CARE

The key leadership contribution of nursing, midwifery and care staff is crucial in maintaining high standards and delivering change.

(Professor Jane Cummings – Chief Nursing Officer, 2016)

NHS England (2014/2015) suggests that quality care is:

[1] Care that is clinically effective
[2] Care that is safe
[3] Care that provides a positive experience for patients

Leadership behaviours are one of the key factors in quality of care. Ensuring care is clinically effective may mean that care is evidence-based, and utilises the latest and most up-to-date methods/technology or treatment. It may mean identifying when practices need to change, or identifying new ways of working for service improvement and helping to trial and lead change. Service improvement requires leadership skills in communication, negotiation and getting people on board to support and manage change.

Care that is safe requires those who deliver it to have integrity and to hold high standards and support others to do the same. In his report *Freedom to Speak Up*, Sir Robert Francis aimed to create conditions for NHS staff to speak out, share good practice and get care providers to make improvements when things go wrong (Francis, 2015). This links very much with transparency and the move towards organisations being assessed by the CQC (Care Quality Commission) on how transparent and open they are. As healthcare workers, we all have a duty, morally and ethically, to speak up and voice concerns if things go wrong. Whistleblowing or reporting concerns is essential for safe care and working environments. This requires not just an awareness that we should speak up when things are going wrong, but who to speak up to. Finally care that provides a positive experience for clients or patients involves auditing the service

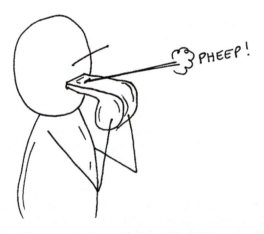

Figure 4.3   Whistleblowing

provided or monitoring patient satisfaction outcomes through patient feedback or complaints. Both practical and personal skills are essential for improving client/patient experience and outcomes.

 Activity 4.2

Think about your current workplace or placement. Are you aware of any policies about raising concerns or whistleblowing? You need to understand your organisation's whistleblowing policies.

- How does the thought of needing to use such policies make you feel?
- What skills and personal qualities do you think would be required when you need to use such policies?

Go Further 4.4

Read this independent review:

Francis, R. (2015) *Freedom to Speak Up: An Independent Review into Creating an Open and Honest Reporting Culture in the NHS* [online]. Available at: http://webarchive.nationalarchives.gov.uk/20150218150343/https://freedomtospeak up.org.uk/wp-content/uploads/2014/07/F2SU_web.pdf

Mentorship

The mentoring and support of workers within healthcare settings is vital to their education and development, and indeed forms an important part of nursing students' competency assessment (NMC, 2016). It is essential for quality of care, and requires many leadership skills. Many organisations now have practice placement mentors who can offer additional support to learners. Mentorship brings with it responsibility, ensuring that the learner is offered support and has access to a wide range of learning experiences. This will require skills in planning and communication when delivering complex learning information; it also considers the need to assess and identify when individual care workers are meeting competencies or identifying where fitness to practise issues may arise.

 Scenario 4.2: Josie

Josie is a care worker and she is helping to support a first year student nurse on a 6-week placement. He is being mentored by one of the qualified nurses on her unit.

She has concerns that she has repeatedly gone over how to take a blood pressure reading and what the readings mean with the student. Other staff members have reported

(Continued)

(Continued)

that the student keeps asking the same questions too, but it is not obvious that these concerns are being tackled.

● How might Josie approach the situation to help support the student?
● Who may Josie speak to/make aware about her concerns?
● What skills might Josie have used in dealing with the situation?

LEADERSHIP QUALITIES AND DEVELOPMENT

Having discussed the current situation in leadership, and why it's important to work toward developing skills in leading, we will now consider what skills or personal qualities may be beneficial in leadership and how these can be developed or promoted.

What leadership skills are required?

Much debate exists on what are the most beneficial and influential skills needed for leadership. These skills are part of a toolbox that you will need, and which ones you use is situation-dependent. This chapter has hopefully allowed you to start thinking about the kind of skills you may require. The next section will look at some key areas for consideration.

The NHS Leadership Academy's most recent model of leadership focuses on nine key areas:

● Inspiring shared purpose
● Leading with care
● Evaluating information
● Connecting our service
● Sharing the vision
● Engaging the team
● Holding to account
● Developing capability
● Influencing for results

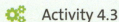 Activity 4.3

Download a copy of the Healthcare Leadership Model from the Leadership Academy from www.leadershipacademy.nhs.uk/wp-content/uploads/dlm_uploads/2014/10/NHSLeadership-LeadershipModel-colour.pdf

In turn, take one of the nine NHS Leadership Academy behaviours:

- In each behaviour, there is a 'What is it not?' section
  - How do you think the 'what it is not' behaviours described occur in practice?
  - What can be done to prevent such behaviours occurring?
- Now look at the 'What it is' section associated with each behaviour
  - How can these behaviours be promoted?

Roebuck (2011) suggests that influencing, decision-making skills, briefing a team, running a task, giving feedback, and learning how to build networks are all key to leadership development. But if we strip away these practical skills, what are the actual skills and tools which some people may inherently have or need to focus on developing?

Communication skills

Developing enhanced verbal communication skills is the backbone to any leadership task. No matter what stage we are at in our careers, we can always remind ourselves to review and reflect on how we verbally communicate with others. Communicating accurately and with an awareness of para-linguistics (tone, pitch, volume) are essential building blocks in verbal communication. Also, you may need to develop your skill at questioning and presenting information to others.

Nonverbal skills are essential. Being able to listen effectively is just as important as being able to convey information. Working on the nonverbal aspects of listening such as eye contact, taking time and using silence is important. Boynton (2009) suggests this can demonstrate physically that you have listened. Active listening is important as it shows respect, and that people are valued; it is also a means of building trust (Battle, 2006). Boynton (2009) suggests this can be demonstrated through not interrupting, and allowing others to finish their sentences. Listening may help you to invest in someone's emotional bank account which is invaluable in collective and transformational leadership styles (Covey, 2004).

🗨 Scenario 4.3   Sarah

The unit manager asks Staff Nurse Sarah to lead on arranging fire safety training for those staff members who are 'out of date' as she is too busy. Sarah starts to compile a list of all the staff on the unit. When she next sees each individual staff member on shift, she asks them 'Are you due your fire training?' Eventually, she manages to ask 10 out of the 13 staff. She wasn't sure if the three staff she hadn't spoken to have had training, so she puts their names down on the training schedule anyway. She sends the list to the training department who keep records of training and who also arrange updates. A few months later, the unit manager asks Sarah why she is still getting reminders about those who are outstanding in their training and some staff have complained that they attended training

(Continued)

(Continued)

before they needed to do so. The unit manager advises she has a spreadsheet with all of the latest updates and that staff should complete this training every three years, Sarah decides to start her list again.

- What questions should Sarah have asked the manager when she was first given this task?
- How should Sarah have communicated with staff and how could she have worded her questions to staff to ensure she got the correct information from them?
- Who else could Sarah have spoken to, to clarify the training schedule?

The above case study highlights the important role communication plays when you are leading on tasks and projects.

Go Further 4.5

The link below is to an RCN (Royal College of Nursing) article on communication skills and has a competency check list:

http://rcnhca.org.uk/top-page-001/communication-methods/verbal-communication/

Emotional intelligence

Goleman et al. (2013) argue that leadership qualities such as developing vision and generating ideas are important, but equally important is the emotional intelligence of leadership. What is emotional intelligence? It can be defined as self-awareness, self-regulation and a level of empathy and understanding of others' perspectives. Having such skills can help to increase positivity and motivation in others and improve our interactions. Frankle (2008) suggests it is the ability to understand and read people's view points and perspectives and put aside glory hunting and ego.

Akerjordet and Severinsson (2008) also suggest that personal emotional intelligence is about self-awareness of your own needs and emotions, and the ability to motivate yourself. Controlling your own emotions in situations helps to overcome difficulties in working with others who have different styles and approaches to your own. Covey (2004) argues that self-awareness and looking after one's own emotional wellbeing is essential in leadership.

Resilience

Resilience can be defined as the ability to recover and bounce back from difficulties or adversities. Much has been written about resilience in childhood studies and in such areas as recovery from trauma and abuse, and examines what makes certain people recover from difficult life situations. Grant and Kinman (2013) argue that the emotional demands of healthcare and being in an environment of constant change requires resilient staff. Whilst some possess natural qualities that help to build resilience, it can also be learned, and that care workers should promote self-care. Further information about resilience can be found in Chapter 11 on mental health and wellbeing.

The personal qualities that add to an individual's resilience are being reflective and self-aware, and having self-confidence. Leaders who are more mindful and self-aware may have better capacity to address complex situations. A key factor in resilience is support mechanisms, such as building good relationships in your team and knowing where to go when advice is needed or when things are difficult.

Resilience is not about taking on too much or not speaking up when you are struggling for fear of being judged as not coping. Therefore, think of resilience as more about building support mechanisms and networks to deal with work issues but not to the extent where the underlying causes are not tackled.

Internal locus of control

Rotter (1990) describes the internal locus of control as 'the degree to which persons expect that reinforcement or an outcome of their behaviour is contingent on their own behaviour or personal characteristics'. People with a high internal locus of control believe in their own ability to control themselves and influence the world around them. They see their future as being in their own hands, and that their own choices can lead to success or failure. West et al. (2015) consider that when what happens around you is under your control, you are motivated to take action to influence events; this is associated with a tendency to be proactive rather than passive. Therefore, developing a focus on situations you have control over can help to eliminate stress and manage the situation more effectively.

 Activity 4.4

Test your resilience at www.robertsoncooper.com/iresilience/

- In which areas are you most resilient?
- In which areas are you less resilient?

Later in the chapter we will look at self-assessment and how you can plan to tackle areas of improvement and promote areas you are strong at in resilience.

POWER

As we move towards a landscape in healthcare where leadership will be more shared and encouraged, you need to understand the role power has in leadership.

The online Oxford Dictionary (2016) defines power as: 'The capacity or the ability to direct or influence the behaviour of others or the course of events'. French and Raven (1959) identified five types of power in a classification that is still relevant today:

- **Legitimate:** Legitimate power could be seen as the type of power that managers have due to position or hierarchy. This comes from the belief that a person has the right to make demands, and to expect others to follow commands. This type of power may have influence to an extent in that people may follow commands that they feel are expected of them for fear of repercussions, but this power may be lost along with position. This is not to say legitimate power is always a negative. Legitimate power if used productively can have great impact by being influential.
- **Reward**: Reward power can be subjective. This type of power seeks compliance from people by offering rewards. This could be a promotion or offering preferential treatment. This type of power can run out if reward promises are not kept, and there is a potential that it could be seen as unethical to offer advantages to a person for carrying out a command. It could be also seen as manipulative.
- **Expert**: Expert power is gained when others may admire or value your knowledge or expertise. Yukl (2012) suggests that expert power is one of the most useful in leadership in getting people on board but expert power does not come overnight and needs to be developed, and trust gained from those who see your expert knowledge as something of value. It is worth noting that expert power can also be lost if those in possession do not maintain their knowledge and trust could be lost along with power if the person seems arrogant or unapproachable with their expert knowledge.
- **Referent:** Referent power is a very different kind of power; it is not commanded by someone's position or title but is gained through an individual's respect or loyalty to that person, often based on personal characteristics. This type of personal power can have great reach and is not easy to achieve. Referent power in leadership is the ability of a leader to gain the respect of others, which is not affected by position or hierarchy (although can be present in those in positions of authority).
- **Coercive**: Coercive power uses the force of an action by use of fear or repercussions if orders are not followed. This type of power may be used in certain circumstances (i.e., in disciplinary meetings) but its use in day-to-day leadership can have a negative effect by using fear to achieve compliance.

The way in which power is used may be interchangeable based on situation and therefore different sources of power may be used in different situations. How power is used may also come across positively or negatively depending on how it is delivered, and this may be in relation to an individual's leadership style or personality. It is important, however, to recognise that being over-reliant on certain types of power may not always gain the best outcome. Activity 4.5 asks you to engage in reflective practice. For more information on how to be reflective, look at Chapter 3, Personal and Professional Development.

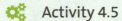

Activity 4.5

Think about some of your current or previous managers or leaders. Thinking about the powers described above, what types of power do you think they used or possessed? What were the good points about that power and how it was used? What were the downsides or when didn't it work well?

LOOKING AFTER YOUR OWN WELLBEING

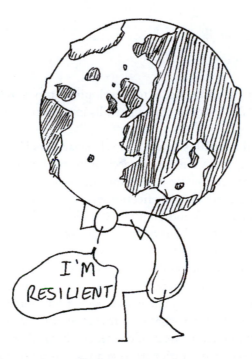

Figure 4.4   Looking after your own wellbeing

Finally, we will focus on a very important factor in personal, professional and leadership development: looking after your own wellbeing (see more detail in Chapter 11, Introduction to Mental Health and Wellbeing). There is much evidence about the value that healthy and motivated staff bring to the quality outcomes of service users in healthcare (Boorman, 2009). Healthcare is challenging, and maintaining a work–life balance is essential. Staff are healthcare's most valuable asset and whilst much is being done to support staff to stay well and healthy in organisations, there are things you can do personally. It is important to consider your own wellbeing as a building block to strong and effective leadership.

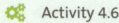

Activity 4.6

Supporting your health: Have a look online at the RCN 'Healthy Workplace Toolkit' at www.rcn.org.uk/professional-development/publications/pub-004964

- What are your thoughts on the toolkit?
- How useful have you found reading it?
- Do you know how to access support for your health and wellbeing? Give examples of where you may seek both physical and mental support inside and outside the workplace.

UNDERSTANDING THE IMPORTANCE OF SELF-ASSESSMENT AND REFLECTION IN LEADERSHIP DEVELOPMENT

Self-assessment is a building block to developing into a reflective practitioner, which is an essential skill in leadership and skills in reflection are required to be able to self-assess.

Rothstein and Burke (2010) suggest that self-awareness is an essential element in leadership. If you want to be effective, especially in healthcare where change is fast paced, you will need to continually learn, grow and adapt. Therefore, self-assessment can be seen as invaluable in personal effectiveness to establish strengths and areas for development in leadership. Jack and Smith (2007) identify that those who truly understand themselves and how their behaviours can impact on others are more self-aware, have more sense of emotional control and stability. Sometimes not enough emphasis is put on concentrating on your strengths, and therefore it could be argued that carrying out self-assessment, recognising strengths and how they could be maximised would be just as important as identifying any challenges. Sometimes, due to work pressures, you do not often get time to consider what your true strengths are and what you do well.

It is still important to identify areas of challenge, things that require improvements or development. Healthcare professionals have a responsibility bound by their professional body to continue to develop and address areas for improvement, especially in light of the reviewed revalidation for nurses and the mandatory need to demonstrate personal development of benefit to practice (NMC, 2015). Healthcare workers are also expected to assess and develop their skills as stated in their code of ethics. Rothstein and Burke (2010) argue that whilst many theorists discuss those born with natural abilities and qualities to lead, through self-assessment, review and feedback, achieving effective leadership skills is within everyone's reach.

Whilst Rothstein and Burke (2010) argue that self-assessment is a building block to advancing individual personal effectiveness, it is also important to understand and appreciate the psychological factors and ethics and morals an individual has as this can often be seen as a factor in leadership styles (Judge and Bono, 2000; Deinert et al., 2015). Therefore completing an online Myers Briggs personality test may be beneficial.

Finally, to evaluate only what you see as strengths and weaknesses may fail to uncover how you are perceived by others. Multi-source feedback processes help you not just to be aware of what you believe are your strengths and weaknesses but what others believe are your strengths and weakness (which may not be the same at all). Jack and Smith (2007) identified in the Johari Window that there is a blind spot, therefore 360-degree feedback is useful for identifying areas you may not have been aware of. The Johari window is a psychological tool created by Luft and Ingham in 1955 as a model to improve self-awareness and personal development. It is a key tool in skill assessment as it encourages openness and a willingness to understand other people's views of your professional strengths and weaknesses. Taking into account the views of others can be a strong motivator to address behaviours to improve leadership practice. It allows the practitioner to demonstrate ownership of their own development.

 Activity 4.7

Research some of the self-assessment tools mentioned here and consider the pros and cons of each method.

Type of assessment tool	Pros	Cons
360° feedback (such as Leadership Academy tool)		
Johari Window		
Personality self-assessment (such as Myers Briggs)		
SWOT		

- 360° feedback: www.leadershipacademy.nhs.uk/resources/healthcare-leadership-model/supporting-tools-resources/healthcare-leadership-model-360-degree-feedback-tool/
- Personality test: www.16personalities.com/free-personality-test
- Johari Window: www.mindtools.com/CommSkll/JohariWindow.htm

IDENTIFYING OPPORTUNITIES FOR LEADERSHIP DEVELOPMENT

Leadership is about drive and innovation, not about seniority

(NHS Plan, 2001)

The final part of this chapter will give ideas for how you could develop your leadership skills both as a health and social care worker and as a student on placement.

Within our own workplaces and educational establishments, there is a wealth of opportunities that allow us to develop a deeper understanding of how the healthcare system works and how leadership skills are used and utilised on a daily basis.

Shadowing senior colleagues and identifying opportunities on placement

Being able to observe what others do is a good learning opportunity to see how others manage a team or how they may deal with difficult situations or competing demands that all require leadership skills. This observation can be informal or formal. Informally, it may be about taking more notice about how others interact. Formally, it may be asking your manager/mentor if you could shadow someone in your organisation or on placement for the day, write up reflective notes later to help you to break down the leadership activities.

Courses and development programmes

Many organisations will have internal courses or programmes that you may be able to access. Try to make yourself aware of the internal continuing professional development opportunities available. There is a wealth of continuing development opportunities through universities, the NHS leadership academy, conferences and annual meetings or local societies. Also you can take free online courses from SCIE, futurelearn, the Open University, and nearly all universities offer free (non-certified) courses.

Social media

Social media can be a useful resource in keeping abreast of current debates in healthcare leadership and most large organisations now have their own Twitter account for example. This can be an easy way of staying up to date with the latest documents and policies and can allow you to become involved in debates (being mindful of any comments you make and how they may be perceived).

Appraisal/IPR

Once you are employed, the identification of development doesn't stop there. An appraisal usually happens annually for employees and allows for the individual to reflect and understand their role and the part they play in their team and organisation. It also allows time to set work objectives for the coming year and discuss achievements from the previous year. It then allows a plan for identifying the knowledge and skills you may need to do your job well and achieve the organisation's objectives and personal development goals. Appraisals are very important for your personal development so utilise them well. Prepare before your appraisal, think about what you might like to be involved in or work towards. As part of this, think about what you will need to do to get to your goal. Appraisal is a great opportunity to discuss with your manager courses you are interested in or opportunities you want to pursue.

Other opportunities

At all levels of your health and social care career, you can look for wider opportunities outside of your placement or employment through volunteering, sitting on boards or acting as advisors. NICE and the CQC are just examples of some of the national organisations who look for those working in healthcare to contribute to their work through sessional or ad hoc work. Students' voices and opinions can be good opportunities for professional development and leadership skill development.

CHAPTER SUMMARY

- We all have the potential, regardless of grade or position in healthcare, to use leadership skills within our roles to ensure quality of care for our clients and patients, whilst also working toward professional and personal development.
- This chapter has introduced the concept of leadership in current healthcare practice.
- Hopefully, the chapter has demystified what leadership may be and given practical direction to how leadership opportunities can be utilised and be developed.

FURTHER READING

The following websites and texts will support your development, knowledge and understanding of leadership and management:

Websites

- The Foundation of Nursing Leadership: www.nursingleadership.org.uk/resources_free.php
- Florence Nightingale Foundation: www.florence-nightingale-foundation.org.uk
- The Health Foundation: www.health.org.uk
- The Kings Fund: www.kingsfund.org.uk
- NHS Employers: www.nhsemployers.org/your-workforce/retain-and-improve/managing-your-workforce/appraisals
- NHS Leadership Academy: www.leadershipacademy.nhs.uk
- Royal College of Nursing: www.rcn.org.uk

Texts

- Ellis, P. and Abbott, J. (2014) Leadership and management skills in health care. *British Journal of Cardiac Nursing*, 9(2): 96–9.
- Grant, L. and Kinman, G. (2013) *The Importance of Emotional Resilience for Staff and Students in the Helping Professions*. York: Higher Education Academy.

- National Skills Academy (2015) *The Leadership Qualities Framework for Adult Social Care.* London: Department of Health/The National Skills Academy.
- NHS England (2016) *Leading Change, Adding Value: A Framework for Nursing, Midwifery and Care Staff.* NHS Publications. Available at: www.england.nhs.uk/wp-content/uploads/2016/05/nursing-framework.pdf.
- NHS Improvement (2016) *Developing People, Improving Care.* Available at: https://improvement.nhs.uk/resources/developing-people-improving-care/.
- Rose, S. (2015) *Better Leadership for Tomorrow.* NHS Leadership Review. London: Department of Health. Available at: www.gov.uk/government/publications/better-leadership-for-tomorrow-nhs-leadership-review.

REFERENCES

Akerjordet, K. and Severinsson, E. (2008) Emotionally intelligent nurse leadership: a literature review study. *Journal of Nursing Management*, 16: 565–77.

Battle, C. (2006) *Effective Listening.* New York: American Society for Training and Development.

Berwick, D. (2013) *A Promise to Learn – A Commitment to Act: Improving the Safety of Patients in England.* London: Department of Health.

Boorman, S. (2009) *NHS Health and Well-Being Review.* London: Department of Health.

Boyatzis, R., Goleman, D. and McKee, A. (2013) *Primal Leadership: Unleashing the Power of Emotional Leadership.* Harvard, MA: Harvard Business Press.

Boynton, B. (2009) How to improve your listening skills. *American Nurse Today*, 4(9): 50–1.

Covey, S.R. (2004) *The 7 Habits of Highly Effective People: Restoring the Character Ethic.* New York: Free Press.

Czabanowska, K., Malho, A., Schröder-Bäck, P., Popa, D. and Burazeri, G. (2014) Do we develop public health leaders? Association between public health competencies and emotional intelligence: a cross-sectional study. *BMC Medical Education*, 14: 83.

Deinert, A., Homan, A., Boer, D., Voelpel, S. and Gutermanna, D. (2015) Transformational leadership sub-dimensions and their link to leaders' personality and performance. *Leadership Quarterly.* doi.org/10.1016/j.leaqua.2015.08.001.

Ellis, P. and Abbott, J. (2014) Leadership and management skills in health care. *British Journal of Cardiac Nursing*, 9(2): 96–9.

Francis, R. (2013) *Report of the Mid Staffordshire NHS Foundation Trust Public Inquiry: Executive Summary.* London: TSO.

Francis, R. (2015) *Freedom to Speak Up: An Independent Review into Creating an Open and Honest Reporting Culture in the NHS.* London: TSO.

Frankle, A. (2008) What leadership styles should senior nurses develop? *Nursing Times*, 104(35): 23–4.

French, J.P.R. and Raven, B.H. (1959) *The Bases of Social Power.* Michigan: University of Michigan, Institute for Social Research.

Goleman, D., Boyatzis, R. and McKee, A. (2013) *Primal Leadership: Unleashing the Power of Emotional Intelligence.* Cambridge, MA: Harvard University Press.

Grant, L. and Kinman, G. (2013) *The Importance of Emotional Resilience for Staff and Students in the Helping Professions.* York: Higher Education Academy.

Griffiths, E.R. (1983) *NHS Management Inquiry.* Available at: www.jstor.org/stable/29512958?seq=1#page_scan_tab_contents (accessed 10 April 2017).

Ham, C. (2014) *Reforming the NHS from Within: Beyond Hierarchy, Inspection and Markets*. London: The Kings Fund.

Health Education England (2015) *Shape of Caring: A Review of the Future Education and Training of Registered Nurses and Care Assistants*. Available at: www.hee.nhs.uk/sites/default/files/documents/2348-Shape-of-caring-review-FINAL.pdf (accessed 17 March 2017).

HSJ Future of NHS Leadership (2015) *Ending the Crisis in NHS Leadership: A Plan for Renewal*. Available at: www.hsj.co.uk/Journals/2015/06/12/y/m/e/HSJ-Future-of-NHS-Leadership-inquiry-report-June-2015.pdf (accessed 17 March 2017).

Jack, K. and Smith, A. (2007) Promoting self-awareness in nurses to improve nursing practice. *Nursing Standard*, 21(32): 47–56.

Judge, T. and Bono, J. (2000) Five factor model of personality and transformational leadership. *Journal of Applied Psychology*, 85(5): 751–65.

Keogh, B. (2013) *Review into the Quality of Care and Treatment Provided by 14 Hospital Trusts in England: Overview Report*. London: NHS England.

Kotter, J. (1996) *Leading Change*. Boston, MA: Harvard Business School Press.

Leggat, S. G. (2007) Effective healthcare teams require effective team members: defining teamwork competencies. *BMC Health Services Research*, 7: 17.

Luft, J. and Ingham, H. (1955) *The Johari Window: A Graphic Model for Interpersonal Relations*. California: University of California Western Training Lab.

NHS England (2014) *Five Year Forward View*. Available at: www.england.nhs.uk/ourwork/futurenhs/ (accessed 17 March 2017).

NHS England (2014/2015) *Annual Review*.

NHS England (2016) *Leading Change, Adding Value: A Framework for Nursing, Midwifery and Care Staff*. Available at: www.england.nhs.uk/wp-content/uploads/2016/05/nursing-framework.pdf (accessed 13 March 2017).

NHS Improvement (2016) *Developing People, Improving Care*. Available at: https://improvement.nhs.uk/resources/developing-people-improving-care/ (accessed 13 March 2017).

NHS Plan (2001) *The NHS Plan: An Action Guide for Nurses, Midwives, and Health Visitors*. Available at: www.nursingleadership.org.uk/publications/agnmhv.pdf (accessed 10 April 2017).

Nursing and Midwifery Council (2015) *The Code: Professional Standards of Practice and Behaviour for Nurses and Midwives*. London: NMC. Available at: www.nmc.org.uk/globalassets/sitedocuments/nmc-publications/nmc-code.pdf (accessed 10 April 2017).

Nursing and Midwifery Council (2016) *Standards for Competence for Registered Nurses*. London: NMC. Available at: www.nmc.org.uk/standards/additional-standards/standards-for-competence-for-registered-nurses/ (accessed 10 April 2017).

Oxford Dictionary (2016) *Power*. Available at: https://en.oxforddictionaries.com/definition/power (accessed 19 June 2017).

Roebuck, C. (2011) *Developing Effective Leadership in the NHS to Maximise the Quality of Patient Care: The Need for Urgent Action*. London: The Kings Fund.

Rose, S. (2015) *Better Leadership for Tomorrow*. NHS Leadership Review. London: Department of Health. Available at: www.gov.uk/government/publications/better-leadership-for-tomorrow-nhs-leadership-review (accessed 19 June 2017).

Rothstein, M.G. and Burke, R.J. (2010) *Self-management and Leadership Development*. London: Edward Elgar.

Rotter, J.B. (1990) Internal vs. external control of reinforcement. *American Psychologist*, 4: 490–3.

The King's Fund (2011) *The Future of Leadership and Management in the NHS: No More Heroes*. London: The King's Fund.

The Kings Fund (2014a) *Culture and Leadership in the NHS*. London: King's Fund.

The Kings Fund (2014b) *Developing Collective Leadership for Health Care*. London: King's Fund.

The Kings Fund (2015) *The Practice of System Leadership: Being Comfortable with Chaos*. London: King's Fund.

Turnbull-James, K. (2011) *Leadership in Context: Lessons from New Leadership Theory and Current Leadership Development Practice*. London: The King's Fund.

West, M., Armit, K., Loewenthal, L., Eckert, R., West, T. and Lee, A. (2015) *Leadership and Leadership Development in Healthcare: The Evidence Base*. London: The King's Fund.

World Health Organization (2009) *Human Factors in Patient Safety Review of Topics and Tools Report for Methods and Measures Working*. Geneva: WHO.

Yukl, G.A. (2012) *Leadership in Organizations*. London: Pearson.

PART TWO

BIOSCIENCES AND ESSENTIAL KNOWLEDGE AND SKILLS FOR CARE

5

BIOSCIENCE

Gillian Rowe

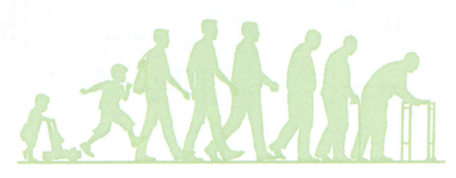

Figure 5.1   The stages of life

This chapter introduces you to the basic anatomy and physiology (A&P) of body systems, and asks you to consider the effects of ageing on the systems and the body as a whole. The immune system is also examined in Chapter 6, Prevention and Control of Infection, and you will use that knowledge to consider the processes involved in wound healing. This chapter links to A&P revision resources to support your learning. Although this chapter does not have a glossary, you will learn plenty of new anatomy and physiology terms through the text and accompanying illustrations.

INTRODUCTION

A good understanding of the anatomy and physiology of the human body is a prerequisite for health and social care workers: you wouldn't take your car to a mechanic who has no idea what happens under the bonnet would you! You need to also understand the changes in the body as it ages, and the impact that ageing has on the various body systems and their functions. When caring for ill people, you need to know what is normal and what is abnormal to assist with the diagnostic process. This chapter gives some

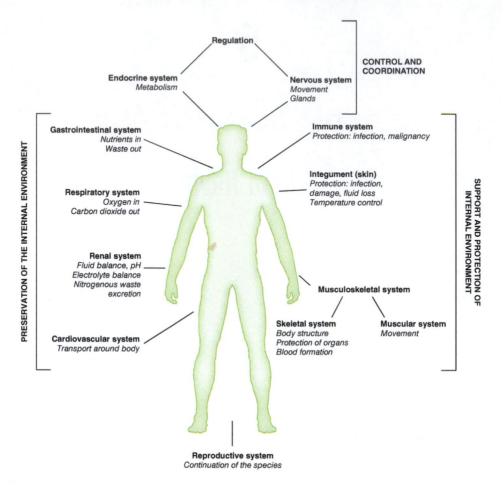

Figure 5.2   Body systems in homeostasis

basic knowledge and indicates where you can go for further information. Remember to watch YouTube channels from reliable sources (NHS, The Khan Academy, Bozeman Science for example) to support your learning.

ANATOMY AND PHYSIOLOGY OF THE BODY SYSTEMS

The digestive system

The digestive system is the process whereby nutrition and hydration is Ingested, Digested, Absorbed, Assimilated and finally, Excreted. The alimentary (or gastrointestinal) canal has several functional adaptations, such as the stomach (Figure 5.4) and the lining of the small intestine to provide the right pH environment for the breakdown and absorption of food (Figure 5.3) and to enable the action of enzymes to complete the process of digestion (see Figure 5.5).

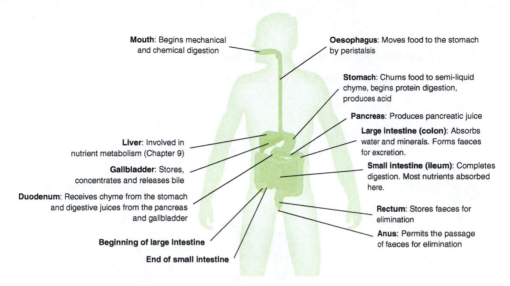

Mouth: Begins mechanical and chemical digestion

Oesophagus: Moves food to the stomach by peristalsis

Stomach: Churns food to semi-liquid chyme, begins protein digestion, produces acid

Pancreas: Produces pancreatic juice

Large intestine (colon): Absorbs water and minerals. Forms faeces for excretion.

Liver: Involved in nutrient metabolism (Chapter 9)

Small intestine (ileum): Completes digestion. Most nutrients absorbed here.

Gallbladder: Stores, concentrates and releases bile

Duodenum: Receives chyme from the stomach and digestive juices from the pancreas and gallbladder

Rectum: Stores faeces for elimination

Anus: Permits the passage of faeces for elimination

Beginning of large Intestine

End of small intestine

Figure 5.3   Components of the digestive system

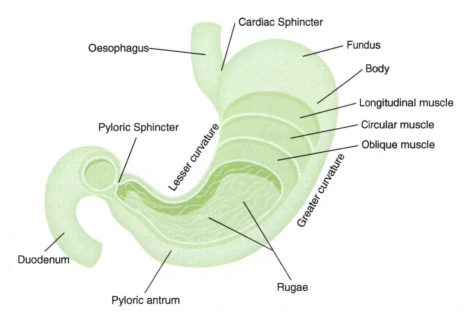

Cardiac Sphincter

Oesophagus

Fundus

Body

Longitudinal muscle

Pyloric Sphincter

Lesser curvature

Circular muscle

Oblique muscle

Greater curvature

Duodenum

Pyloric antrum

Rugae

Figure 5.4   The stomach

Understanding the function of enzymes is crucial to your understanding of the system. Enzymes function best at 36–37°C, which is why homeostasis maintains your body at this constant. If your temperature is lower, fewer reactions occur, if it is higher, enzyme proteins become denatured (this means change shape) and cannot function through the lock and key mechanism (see Figure 5.5).

Go Further 5.1

Check out the following online document to find out more about enzymes:

http://biologymad.com/resources/EnzymesRevision.pdf

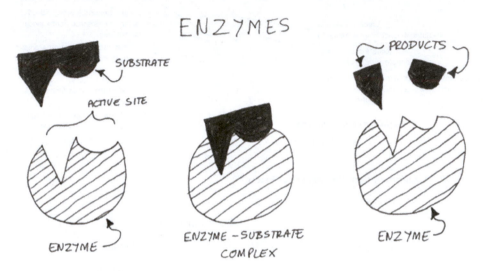

Figure 5.5   Enzymes lock and key

When the immune system responds to attack by producing eicosanoid prostaglandins (to kill invaders) which elevate the temperature (producing fever), the immune system is at odds with the digestive system as homeostatic mechanisms try to reduce temperature – you can see this when charting the temperature of someone with an infection: the immune system pushes the temperature up and homeostasis tries to bring it down, hence the spikes on the chart.

Once the enzymes have broken food into its constituent particles, absorption takes place through the gut lining. Finger-like projections called villi vastly increase the surface area to speed the process up; sugars and proteins are absorbed by the capillaries and sent to the liver via the hepatic portal system and fats are absorbed via the lacteals of the villi (see Figure 5.6). At this stage fat is in the form of chylomicrons and enters the circulatory system via the lymphatic system at the thoracic duct and empties into the subclavian vein.

The large intestine has only minor absorptive function other than reclaiming water and salts (anyone who has had diarrhoea will know how effective it is); it does, however, absorb vitamins which are created by bowel flora, such as vitamin K, vitamin B12, thiamine and riboflavin. This vitamin creation is essential for those with poor diet but the producing bacteria can be killed by antibiotics. Compacted waste is then excreted.

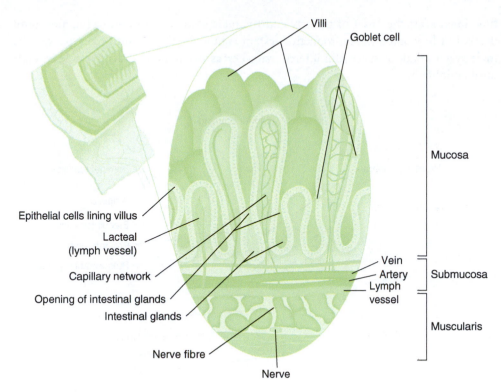

Villi
Goblet cell
Mucosa
Epithelial cells lining villus
Lacteal
(lymph vessel)
Capillary network
Vein
Artery
Lymph
vessel
Submucosa
Opening of intestinal glands
Intestinal glands
Muscularis
Nerve fibre
Nerve

Figure 5.6   Structure of the small intestine

Effects of ageing on the digestive system

As the person ages, taste bud replacement lessens (which is why older people claim modern food is tasteless), slowing peristalsis increases constipation and the likelihood of developing haemorrhoids, absorption slows, which taken with loss of taste buds, difficulties with chewing and constipation can lead to older folks suffering from loss of appetite and poor nutrition. Some drugs are absorbed through the lining of the colon and the condition of the ageing gut will have an impact on how effective their uptake is.

Go Further 5.2

Read through this online document about the digestive system:

www.lamission.edu/lifesciences/lecturenote/aliphysio1/digestion.pdf

The reproductive system

Reproduction is crucial for the survival of any species and ours is no different. It could be argued that the basic purpose of our species is to reproduce. The equipment that differentiates men and women biologically is our reproductive organs. They become functional after the onset of puberty and the male system continues to function until death, but in women the reproductive system is functional only until menopause. The male system ends at successful intercourse whereas women's reproductive role extends until childbirth.

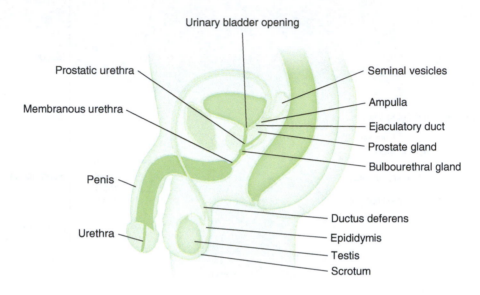

Figure 5.7   The male reproductive system

The functions of the male reproductive organs (Figure 5.7) are the production of male gametes (spermatozoa), the transportation of sperm to the female reproductive tract and production of the male sex hormone testosterone, which controls the secondary male sexual characteristics (body and facial hair, male physique, vocal chords).

The functions of the female reproductive organs (Figure 5.8) are to produce eggs (ova), transport the ova to the uterus (via the fallopian tubes) and provide an environment for a growing fetus. If the ova is not fertilised, the lining of the uterus is shed (menstruation). The ovaries also produce the hormones oestrogen and progesterone under the direction of follicle stimulating hormone, produced by the pituitary gland. Under the influence of human chorionic gonadotrophin, oestrogen and progesterone produced in the ovary (corpus luteum) maintain pregnancy until the placenta is mature enough to produce its own hormones.

Both the vagina and the uterus are potential spaces, this means that they are able to stretch to accommodate the growing baby and to allow passage of the baby into the world. As the baby grows, so does the uterus (see Figure 5.9). The developing child is supported by nutrition and oxygen from its mother via the placenta and umbilical cord (see Figure 5.9). Whilst they do not share blood supply, products pass through the mother's blood and diffuse (or are actively transported) across the placental barrier to the child. Carbon dioxide and waste products are passed back to the mother using the same system.

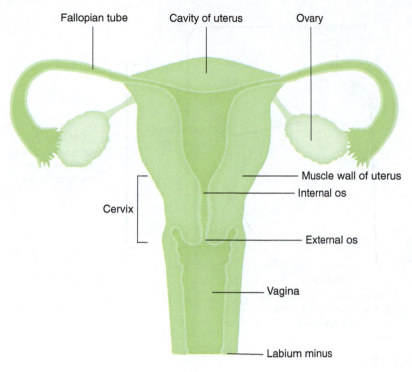

Fallopian tube

Cavity of uterus

Ovary

Muscle wall of uterus

Internal os

Cervix

External os

Vagina

Labium minus

Figure 5.8   The female reproductive system

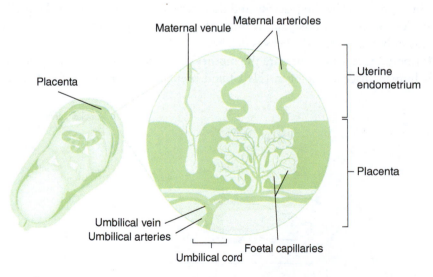

Maternal venule

Maternal arterioles

Placenta

Uterine endometrium

Placenta

Umbilical vein

Umbilical arteries

Umbilical cord

Foetal capillaries

Figure 5.9   Pregnancy

As the birth approaches, oestrogen levels peak, causing intrauterine ripples called Braxton Hicks (false labour), this causes the endometrium to create receptors for oxytocin (see Figure 5.10) which are secreted by the foetal cells. The hypothalamus

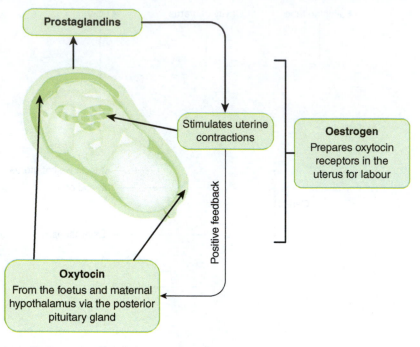

Figure 5.10   Birth

gland also cascades oxytocin and this produces rhythmic contractions in the uterus. Relaxin is produced by the placenta and this increases the flexibility of the pelvic ligaments. As the contractions gain in force, the mucus plug gives way (the show), the cervix is fully dilated and the baby is delivered.

Hormonal interactions prepare the mother's body for lactation – the placenta produces human placenta lactogen (HPL) and prepares the breasts for lactation, HPL

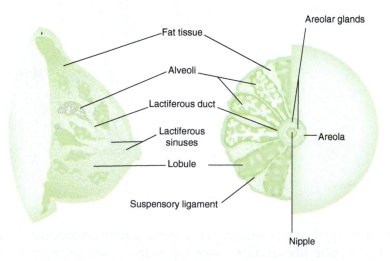

Figure 5.11   Lactation

triggers the hypothalamus to excrete prolactin releasing hormones (PRH) which then stimulates the pituitary gland to make prolactin (Figure 5.11). While this process is going on (about 36 hours), the mammary glands produce colostrum, an essential vitamin-rich pre-milk which contains antibodies, antimicrobial factors and growth hormones to protect and stimulate the new baby.

Effects of ageing on the reproductive system

Men retain their ability to reproduce into extreme old age; however, the rate of sperm production slows although sperm numbers remain the same. There may be an increase in chromosomal abnormalities. The skin pouches that hold the testicles continue to grow under the effect of declining testosterone, leading to sagging; also the prostate gland enlarges.

Women undergo menopause at ages 45–55, although the use of hormone replacement therapy can push this age back until well into the 60s. At menopause, the production of oestrogen in the ovaries decreases by about 95% and there is a rapid decline in oocytes. Breasts tissue loses elasticity leading to sag and the vaginal walls become thinner and lose elasticity, leading to an increased risk of prolapse.

Go Further 5.3

Read the following chapter notes on the reproductive system:

www.gallantsbiocorner.com/uploads/9/1/3/5/9135671/sexnotes.pdf

---

The urinary system

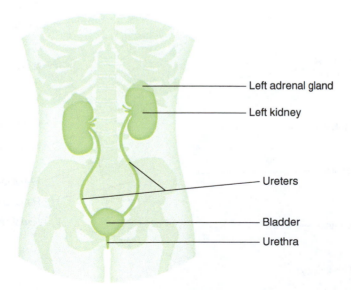

Figure 5.12   The urinary system

Adult humans consist of 60% fluid, although content varies with age: a newborn has about 80% water whereas in elderly people it can be as low as 50%. Table 5.1 shows how fluid is distributed throughout the body

Table 5.1   Body fluid

The greatest part of the fluid is found in the cells (known as intracellular fluid)	about 25 litres
The rest is extracellular fluid (outside the cells and is made up of interstitial or tissue fluid), fluid that bathes the cells and is in the spaces between the cells	about 10 litres
Blood plasma (in blood vessels known as intravascular fluid)	about 3 litres
Urine and fluid in bowel	about 1.5 litres

How much liquid is that?

The urinary system comprises of two kidneys, two ureters connected to one bladder and one urethra which is the outgoing tube (see Figure 5.12). The function of the urinary system is the elimination of waste metabolites and the control of the salt/water balance (osmoregulation). The kidneys (see Figure 5.13) filter all the circulating blood in the body 300 times a day. The function of the kidneys can be summarised as:

- Filtration
- Absorption
- Elimination

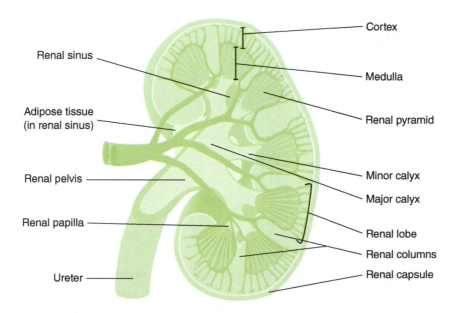

Figure 5.13   The kidneys

Kidneys clean blood and tissue fluid by removing excess water and urea which are excreted in urine. Urea, which gives urine its name, is a nitrogen-containing substance produced in the liver to remove excess amino acids. Sugar and mineral products are reabsorbed for reuse in the body.

Regulation of water is a homeostatic mechanism which controls the movement of water in and out of cells by osmosis and by receptor cells in the blood informing the hypothalamus in the brain if blood is too thick. The brain responds through the pituitary gland by producing antidiuretic hormone (arginine vasopressin) which prevents dehydration by conserving body fluids through reabsorbing dilute urine and triggering the sensation of thirst. Too much fluid in the body (hypovolemia) can be caused by congestive cardiac failure (oedema), kidney failure, liver disease (ascites), acquired brain injury, or through iatrogenic causes such as saline intravenous fluid overload.

Go Further 5.4

For further detail of the urinary system visit www.pearsonhighered.com/content/dam/one-dot-com/one-dot-com/us/en/higher-ed/en/products-services/course-products/amerman-1e-info/pdf/amerman-sample-chapter24.pdf

---

Effects of ageing on the urinary system

Kidney tissue decreases along with a concomitant loss of renal nephrons, the blood vessels supplying the kidneys can suffer from atherosclerosis (hardening) with risk of aneurysm. The bladder muscles can weaken leading to incontinence, the loss of muscle tone can lead to a displaced urethra, and in men the enlarged prostate can cause flow pressure issues and retention. Retention in both men and women can lead to urinary tract infections (UTIs) which are difficult to resolve. The use of in-dwelling catheters is now discouraged unless absolutely essential as they are known to promote UTIs and subsequent kidney disease.

The integumentary system

Skin is the body's boundary between the internal and external world: it is the first line of defence of the immune system as it contains a whole biome of commensal (helpful) bacteria; it contains nerve endings that inform the brain about the external world; it protects against dehydration (by waterproofing), against overheating (sweat glands) and against sunburn (melanin) (see Figure 5.14). The integumentary system is the largest system of the body; in an adult, averagely, the skin has a surface of 1.5 to 2 square meters (22 square feet or about the same area of a single sized bed) and would weigh (approximately) 9.7 kg (or 20lb). The thickness of the skin varies, being thinnest in your eyelids and thickest on the soles of your feet. The skin has three layers (Table 5.2).

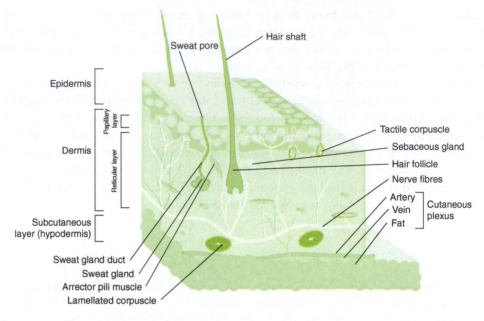

Figure 5.14   The integumentary system

The skin is an organ of regulation in that it aids homeostatic mechanisms of thermoregulation and osmoregulation. It also acts as a reservoir for the synthesis of vitamin D. Skin is also an organ of sensation – cold, heat, touch and pain. Wounds to the skin affect all the skin functions, especially burns or wounds that lead to scarring.

Table 5.2   The layers of the skin

The epidermis	A sheet of dead cells that forms a protective barrier made of squamous cells which originate in the basal layer of the dermis and move up to the epidermis. The epidermis also contains Langerhans cells, keratinocytes and melanocytes and the hair follicles
The dermis	Contains sebaceous glands (which secrete sebum which is made of cholesterol, fatty acids and waxy esters), arrector pili muscles, blood vessels, nerve endings, sweat glands and lymphatic channels
The subcutaneous fatty layer	Nerve fibres and Pacinian (lamellar) corpuscles that sense vibratory pressure

Effects of ageing on the integumentary system

Skin becomes more fragile with age. It loses collagen and elastin (elastosis); solar elastosis is the weather-beaten appearance of older people who work outdoors. Melanocyte production slows and the skin becomes translucent. Large pigmented spots appear on skin exposed to the sun (liver spots). The blood vessels of the dermis become more fragile leading to frequent bruising (senile purpura). The sebaceous glands produce less sebum resulting in the skin drying as oil production decreases. The subcutaneous layer retains less fat which reduces insulation and means that older people feel the cold and are at greater risk of hyperthermia. Fat loss and mobility limiting musculoskeletal disorders increases the risk of decubitus (pressure) ulcers for ageing skin. If this is complicated by type 2 diabetes, wound healing time rises by a factor of 4.

Go Further 5.5

A good chapter to read for further detail on the integumentary system can be found here: www.lamission.edu/lifesciences/AliAnat1/Chap%203%20-%20 Integumentary%20System.pdf

---

The cardiovascular system

The cardiovascular system is comprised of the heart and vascular tubing (blood vessels). Figure 5.15 shows the thoracic cavity showing the position of the heart and lungs.

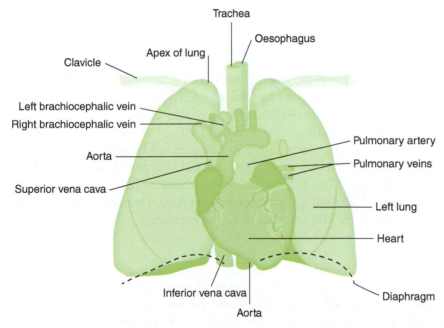

Figure 5.15   The heart and lungs

The cardiac system

The heart is a double pump: the upper chambers (atria, meaning waiting area from the Latin *atrium*) contract first, forcing blood into the two lower chambers, the ventricles (Figure 5.16). Ventricular force is higher as the blood has further to go and this is

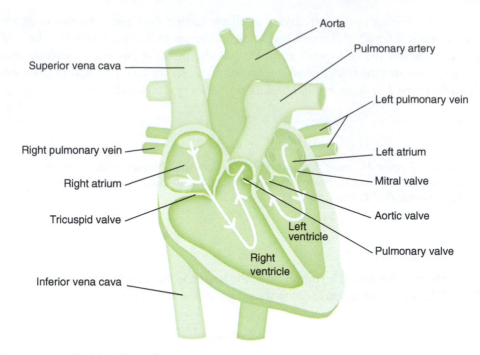

Figure 5.16   The blood flow of the heart

evidenced by the anatomy of the heart, where ventricular muscle is very thick compared to the upper heart. Blood is prevented from back flow by valves between the chambers and at the end of the blood vessels (see Figure 5.16).

The heart is powered by action potentials initiated at the sinoatrial node (cardiac pacemaker) and conducted to left atrium via Bachmann's bundle causing atrial contraction, the signal then travels to the atrioventricular node which propagates the current through the Bundle of His to the Purkinje fibres which causes ventricular contraction (see Figure 5.17). The resting heart rate (sinus rhythm) is between 60 and 100 beats per minute and can exceed 200 beats per minute at exercise.

The vascular system

Deoxygenated venous blood is returned to the right side of the heart, oxygenated blood from the lungs is cycled via the left side of the heart. Venous blood travels through veins, back flow is prevented by lumen (which can become less effective with age and occupation becoming varicose). Arterial blood travels through arteries, the largest of which is the aorta (see Figure 5.16). Arteries have a thick muscular wall which allows for expansion to accommodate the 70–90 millilitres of blood ejected. See Figure 5.18 to examine the structural difference between arteries and veins.

Vessels become smaller the further away they are from the heart (arterioles, venules) until they become hair-like single-cell-thick capillaries, which is where gas

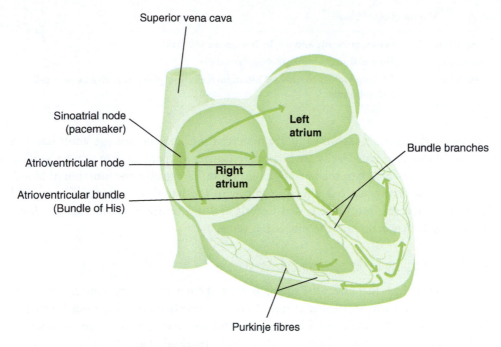

Superior vena cava

Sinoatrial node
(pacemaker)

Left
atrium

Atrioventricular node

Bundle branches

Right
atrium

Atrioventricular bundle
(Bundle of His)

Purkinje fibres

Figure 5.17   The cardiac electrical system

(and nutrient/waste) exchange takes place, with oxygen diffusing out and carbon dioxide diffusing in (internal respiration).

Blood is made up of (approximately) 55% plasma and 45% cells (erythrocytes, leucocytes and platelets). The volume of blood occupied by the cells is called the haematocrit. Plasma is made up of 92% water, 7% plasma proteins (albumin, globulin,

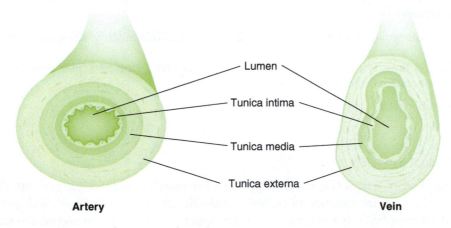

Lumen

Tunica intima

Tunica media

Tunica externa

Artery

Vein

Figure 5.18   Structure of arteries and veins

Table 5.3   The function of blood

Transportation	Gases, nutrients and waste, hormones and heat
Regulation	Temperature, osmoregulation, blood pH
Protection	Clotting factors to prevent blood loss; micro-organisms such as white cells and antibodies

fibrinogen: the clotting factors) and 1% dissolved solutes. The average adult has 5–6 litres of blood. Red blood cells are biconcave (saucer shaped) to give greater surface area for oxygen to attach to the haemoglobin. Table 5.3 explains the function of blood.

The circulatory system has a relationship with the lymphatic system. Tissue fluid (lymph) is collected into blind-ended lacteals and is a return route to the blood, via lymph vessels that drain into the subclavian veins.

The effects of ageing on the cardiovascular system

Most of the changes that affect the ageing heart and circulatory system are as a result of disease. By late adulthood, cardiac output decreases and cholesterol increases leading to blood vessel walls thickening and hardening (arteriosclerosis), which reduces elasticity in the arteries and increases blood pressure (hypertension). More blood is left in the ventricles, decreasing ejection fraction to below 70%, and the heart rate may slow due to loss of pacemaker cells, leading to loss of capacity at the major organs. Heart murmurs increase as the cardiac valves become less flexible. Functional blood volume decreases and baroreceptors that monitor blood pressure when you change position become less sensitive, which can cause orthostatic hypotension.

Go Further 5.6

Download the following PDF which details the cardiovascular system and blood circulation:

www.biologymad.com/resources/Ch%206%20-The%20Circulatory%20System.pdf

Visit the British Heart Foundation website to read about cardiovascular diseases, current research and preventative measures:

www.bhf.org.uk

The respiratory system

The respiratory system (Figure 5.19) provides the route for entry of oxygen into the body and a route for excretion of carbon dioxide. Breathing warms or cools and moistens the atmospheric air and it cleans the atmospheric air using mucus and cilia to trap airborne particles.

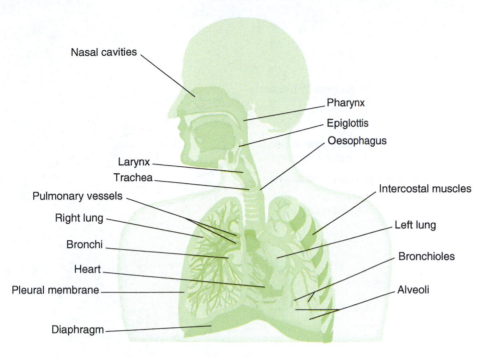

Figure 5.19   The structure of the respiratory system

The human lungs are a pair of large, spongy organs optimised for gas exchange between our blood and the air. They are lobular, with three on the right side and two on the left (space needed to accommodate the heart). Our bodies require oxygen in order to survive and the lungs provide us with vital oxygen while also removing carbon dioxide before it can reach hazardous levels. Air is drawn in through the mouth or nose and passes through the nasal or buccal cavity, pharynx and larynx, drawn down through the trachea into the right and left bronchus and thence to the alveoli (Figure 5.20). Table 5.4 details other functions of the respiratory system. Figure 5.21 explains to the mechanics of breathing.

Gas exchange takes place in the alveoli of the lungs. Inspired atmospheric air contains 78% nitrogen, 21% oxygen, 0.04% carbon dioxide and variable amounts of water vapour. Expired air contains 78% nitrogen, 14% oxygen, 4% carbon dioxide and is saturated with water vapour. Once oxygen has diffused into the bloodstream it binds to oxyhaemoglobin molecules (HbO_2) in the red blood cells. The actual number of O_2 molecules binding depends upon the partial pressure (PO_2) of oxygen. See Figure 5.22 for detail of gas exchange.

Control of breathing is coordinated in the brain as respiratory rate has a relationship with the heart rate. The respiratory centre is in the medulla oblongata, which is responsible for inspiration, basic respiratory rhythm and forced expiration. The pneumotaxic centre in the pons varolli is responsible for inhibition of inspiration, which results in

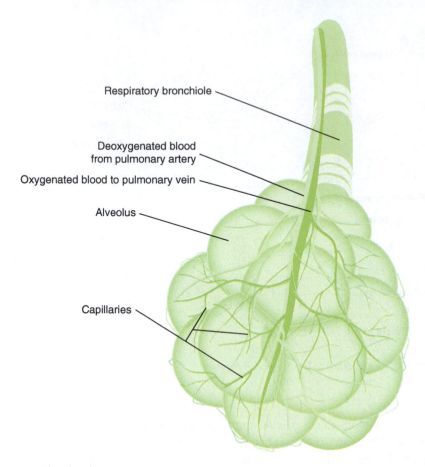

Respiratory bronchiole

Deoxygenated blood from pulmonary artery

Oxygenated blood to pulmonary vein

Alveolus

Capillaries

Figure 5.20   The alveoli

Table 5.4   Other functions of the respiratory system

Hearing	The auditory tube extends from the nasopharynx to the middle ear and protects the tympanic membrane
Protection	Lymphatic tissue protecting the tonsils (pharyngeal and laryngeal), cough reflex, mucus escalator to trap and remove particles
Speech	The thoracic cavity acts as a resonating chamber for volume, pitch and intonation

expiration. The mechanical action of breathing is under control of the central nervous system. Innervation of the diaphragm is by the phrenic nerve (which originates from the C3, C4 and C5) and innervation of the external intercostal muscles is by the intercostal nerves (which originate from the thoracic portion of the spinal cord T1–T12) (see Figure 5.23).

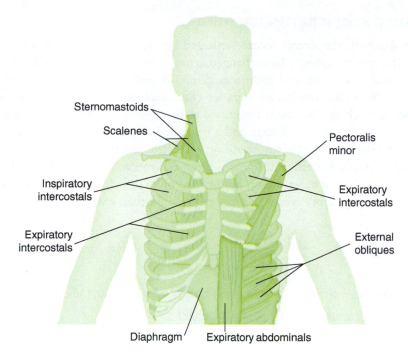

The mechanics of breathing

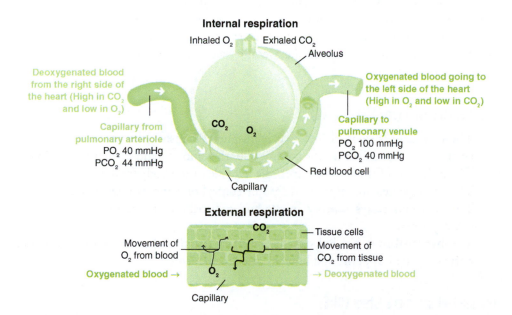

Internal respiration

Inhaled O_2 Exhaled CO_2

Alveolus

Deoxygenated blood
from the right side of
the heart (High in CO_2
and low in O_2)

Oxygenated blood going to
the left side of the heart
(High in O_2 and low in CO_2)

CO_2 O_2

Capillary from
pulmonary arteriole
PO_2 40 mmHg
PCO_2 44 mmHg

Capillary to
pulmonary venule
PO_2 100 mmHg
PCO_2 40 mmHg

Red blood cell

Capillary

External respiration

CO_2 Tissue cells

Movement of
O_2 from blood

Movement of
CO_2 from tissue

Oxygenated blood → O_2 → Deoxygenated blood

Capillary

Figure 5.22   Internal and external respiration

The effects of ageing on the respiratory system

The air spaces in the alveoli become enlarged and lose their elasticity, meaning that there is less area for gases to be exchanged across. The lungs become stiffer (lose compliance), muscle strength and endurance diminish, and the chest wall becomes rigid. The strength of the respiratory muscles (the diaphragm and intercostal muscles) decreases. This change is closely connected to the general health of the person. There is an increase in mucus production and a decrease in the activity and number of cilia. Older people cough more to remove airborne particles and to clear the lungs of phlegm. The body becomes less efficient in monitoring and controlling breathing. All of these changes mean that an older person might have more difficulty coping with increased stress on their respiratory system, such as pneumonia, than a younger person would.

Go Further 5.7

To find out more on human respiratory system physiology, read the online document:

www.liverpool.ac.uk/~gdwill/hons/gul_lect.pdf

The nervous system

The nervous system is multifunctional: it allows you to speak, hear, feel, sense, taste, see, smell, think, create, respond, move, have morals, experience pain and pleasure, learn and remember. It has two main parts: the central nervous system (the brain and spinal cord) and the peripheral nervous system (autonomic, somatic, sympathetic and parasympathetic nervous systems).

The cranial cavity (see Figure 5.24)

- The cerebrum is divided into two hemispheres housing the motor and sensory cortex. It is responsible for the control of both voluntary and involuntary actions.
- The right side of the brain controls the left side of the body (and vice versa).
- The basal ganglia are responsible for fine control of complex movements.
- The thalamus relays sensory inputs and redistributes them to the appropriate sensory areas.
- The hypothalamus has links to the pituitary gland and controls the autonomic nervous system, appetite and homeostatic mechanisms.

The central nervous system (CNS)

The spinal cord runs from the brain to the lumbar region and is protected by the vertebrae. It contains cerebrospinal fluid which circulates within membranes (meninges)

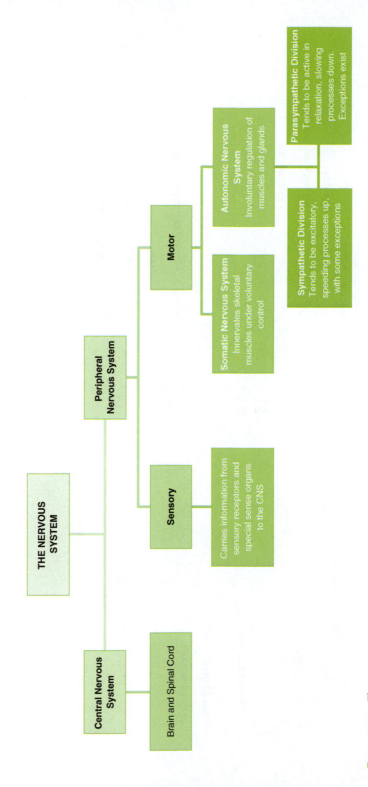

Figure 5.23   The nervous system

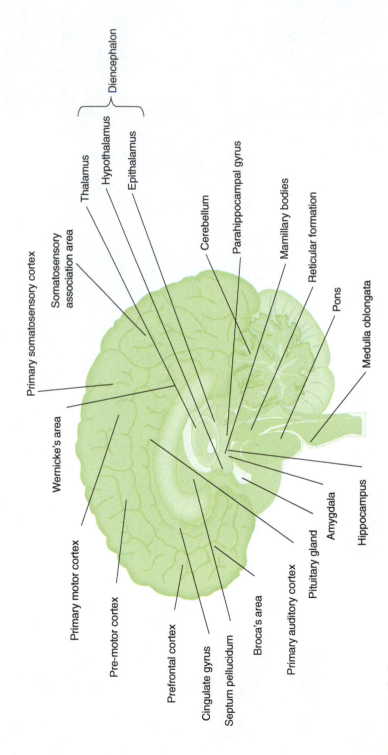

Figure 5.24   The brain

Diencephalon
- Thalamus
- Hypothalamus
- Epithalamus

Primary somatosensory cortex

Somatosensory association area

Cerebellum

Parahippocampal gyrus

Mamillary bodies

Reticular formation

Pons

Medulla oblongata

Wernicke's area

Primary motor cortex

Pre-motor cortex

Prefrontal cortex

Cingulate gyrus

Septum pellucidum

Broca's area

Primary auditory cortex

Pituitary gland

Amygdala

Hippocampus

around the outside of the CNS and also inside a canal within the CNS. Both the brain and spinal cord contain white matter which contains axons and dendron, and grey matter which is mainly the cell bodies of neurons. The brain stem links the spinal cord to the brain and attaches to the medulla oblongata which controls and coordinates three vital centres: the cardiovascular centre, the respiratory centre and the reflex centres for vomiting, coughing, sneezing and swallowing.

The peripheral nervous system

This has several parts: there are nerves that control the involuntary (autonomic) activities of the body, such as the heart beat or digestion, and nerves that control voluntary activities of the body, such as musculoskeletal movement. The autonomic nervous system controls the sympathetic system, better known as 'fight and flight': the effects on the smooth muscles of the airways, blood vessels, cardiac muscle and various glands are rapid; the parasympathetic nervous system resets the body to default after the excitement has calmed down.

Nerve structure and function

Nerve cells are called neurons and they come in three shapes and sizes, depending on their function (see Figure 5.25 and Table 5.5). Sensory neurons send messages moving away from a central organ or point and relay messages from receptors (such as in the skin) **to** the brain or spinal cord. Interneurons are relay neurons and relay messages from sensory neurons to motor neurons. Motor neurons send messages towards a central organ or point and relay messages **from** the brain or spinal cord to the muscles and organs.

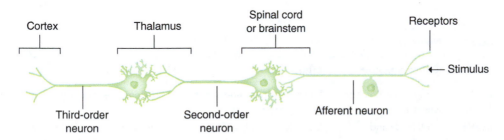

Figure 5.25   A sensory neuron

Each neuron has a cell body and axons and dendrites. Messages are relayed along the branches by action potentials which are controlled by the Schwann cells and the nodes of Ranvier. These are protected by a wrapping of myelin sheath. Neurons are complex and do not reproduce once damaged, they cannot heal or be repaired, although science is doing its very best to overcome this. Neurons and nerve endings do not actually touch each other;

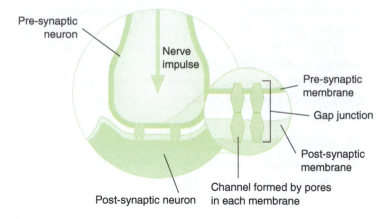

Figure 5.26   The synapse

there is a slight gap called a synapse (see Figure 5.26). Messages need to pass across the synapse and they do this via hormones called neurotransmitters which travel across the synapse and lock into receptor sites and thus pass on the action potential.

Pre-synaptic neuron = neuron sending impulse

Post-synaptic neuron = neuron receiving impulse

Go Further 5.8

This process is quite complex; you might improve your understanding of this by watching Bozeman Science or Khan Academy YouTube videos.

Table 5.5   Neurons

	Sensory neuron	Interneuron	Motor neuron
Length of fibre	Long dendrites and short axon	Short dendrites and short or long axon	Short dendrites and long axons
Location	Cell body and dendrite are outside of the spinal cord	Entirely within the CNS	Dendrites and the cell body are located in the spinal cord; the axon is outside of the spinal cord
Function	Conducts impulse to the spinal cord	Interconnects the sensory neuron with appropriate motor neuron	Conducts impulse to an effector (muscle or gland)

Nerves are made up of hundreds of neurons somewhat analogous to an electrical cable made up of hundreds of filaments. They form the nerve pathways; some are

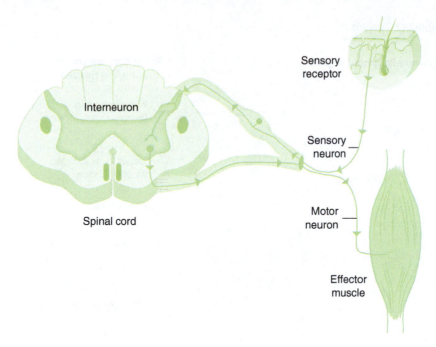

Figure 5.27   The reflex arc

simple reflexes, which are innate, such as blinking or knee jerk (Figure 5.27), and some are learned responses and require conscious thought; these are very complex as different responses can result from a single stimulus.

Effects of ageing on the nervous system

With ageing there is a loss of nerve/brain cells which do not regenerate, and coupled with lessening production of neurotransmitters this leads to increases in reaction time. Receptors become less sensitive, which results in reduced sense of touch and sensitivity to pain. Changes in memory and increased forgetfulness may be the result of disease processes such as dementias, but cognitive decline generally depends on the individual. Keeping intellectually active can slow decline, although research (studies too numerous to mention individually) evidences that older adults perform less well on tasks involving encoding, retention and retrieval of information.

Go Further 5.9

Read more on the nervous system:

www.blackwellpublishing.com/intropsych/pdf/chapter3.pdf

The immune system

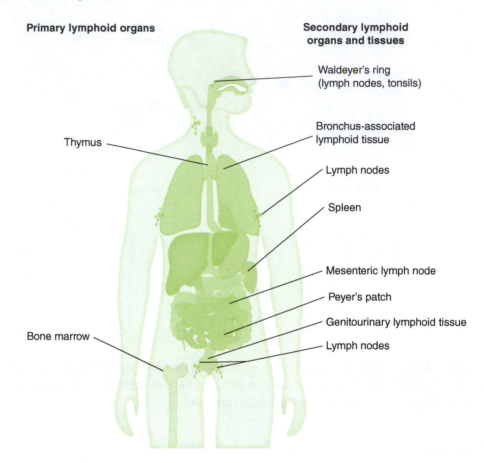

Primary lymphoid organs

Thymus

Bone marrow

Secondary lymphoid organs and tissues

Waldeyer's ring (lymph nodes, tonsils)

Bronchus-associated lymphoid tissue

Lymph nodes

Spleen

Mesenteric lymph node

Peyer's patch

Genitourinary lymphoid tissue

Lymph nodes

Figure 5.28   The immune system

You have on average about one hundred thousand bacteria on every square centimetre of your skin. These dine on the 10 billion flakes of skin that you shed every day, plus all the oils and minerals that you secrete. There are trillions more inside your body – in your nose, in your gut (more trillions) – they can reproduce in less than 10 minutes, so in 24 hours one can become 280,000 billion. However, we cannot live without bacteria; they process wastes, synthesise vitamins and go to war against invading microbes. Table 5.6 introduces you to the words we use to describe types of infective agents.

Table 5.6   Infective agents

Vector	Living organisms that can transmit infectious diseases between humans or from animals to humans
Pathogen	An infective agent such as a bacteria, virus, fungus or parasite
Antigen	A chemical constituent of a pathogen, which the immune system recognises as a threat

You can find more detail about the immune system in Chapter 6 on the prevention and control of infection.

The immune system works across the body systems because bacteria, fungi, viruses and parasites enter through orifices such as the mouth, nose, ears, genitals, eyes and skin pores and through wounds, cuts and abrasions and can affect every part of the body. The immune system can override homeostasis and is known as the 'command and control' system (see Figure 5.29). There are three parts to the immune system, we will look at them in turn.

The first lines of defence

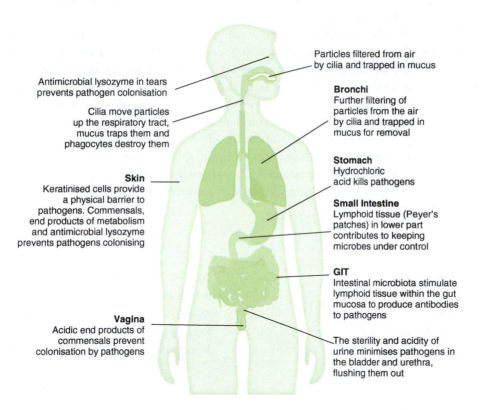

Figure 5.29 The first lines of defence

- The skin: prevents pathogens entering the body and has a biome of helpful commensal bacteria.
- The nose and bonchi: contain sticky mucus that traps pathogens; they are coughed up and swallowed. Macrophages (phagocytes) swim in the fluid that surrounds the alveoli, these eat and destroy invading microbes. When they have achieved their task, they too are swept up the bronchi via the mucus escalator.
- Blood: contains histamines to invoke the inflammatory response.

- Tears and saliva: contain the killer enzyme lysosome.
- The stomach: gastric acid has a pH of 1.5, this kills many pathogens.

The second lines of defence: the non-specific or innate system

The second line of defence is the non-specific immune system. This can kill or limit the spread of pathogens, but it is not an efficient killer of specific invaders as it does not learn to recognise one particular antigen from another. This line of defence uses engulfing cells called phagocytes, which are cells that eat invading organisms (think Pacman). These are the link between the non-specific and specific immune system. Once a phagocyte has engulfed the invader, it becomes an antigen-presenting cell, which then stimulates the mediated system.

Inflammation is one of the first responses of the immune system to infection. The symptoms of inflammation are redness and swelling, which are caused by increased blood flow into a tissue (which is what actually causes the pain). Inflammation is produced by the mast cells eicosanoids and cytokines, which are released by injured or infected cells. Eicosanoid prostaglandins produce fever and the dilation of blood vessels associated with inflammation, and leukotrienes that attract leucocytes.

Leucocytes are the main defence in the bloodstream; they float through the stream until they detect the chemical signals of an invader, then travel to the cells to mount an inflammatory response (chemotaxis). They are either granular or agranular depending on the presence of small grain-like vesicles in their cytoplasm. Table 5.7 gives the different types of leucocytes.

Table 5.7   Leucocytes

Monocytes	Turn into macrophages and engulf invaders
Neutrophils	Attack and kill bacteria and fungi
Eosinophils	Kill parasites such as flatworms and flukes
Eicosanoids	Prostaglandins which cause fever
Basophils	Release histamine during allergic reactions

Cytokines

These are chemical messengers that carry communication between cells and include:

- interleukins that are responsible for communication between white blood cells, and
- interferons that have anti-viral effects, such as shutting down protein synthesis in the host cell.

These cytokines and other chemicals recruit immune cells to the site of infection and promote healing following the removal of pathogens.

The complement system is a biochemical cascade that attacks the surfaces of foreign cells. It contains over 20 different proteins and is named for its ability to 'complement'

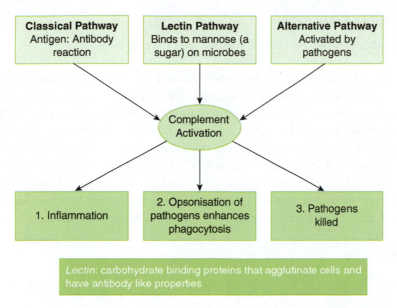

Figure 5.30   Detail of complement activation

the killing of pathogens by antibodies. Complement is the major humoral component of the nervous system/innate immune response (see Figure 5.30).

The third line of defence or the adaptive response system

Lymphocytes are specialised attack cells which respond to both external and internal (for instance cancer) invaders. They are an improvised response to a specific invader and are created in the bone marrow. They are capable of remembering invaders. This defence system is slower to react as it must determine the nature of the attack and formulate a response. Although mature lymphocytes look pretty much alike, they are extraordinarily diverse in their functions.

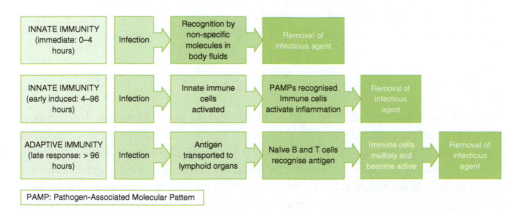

Figure 5. 31   Schematic of the three systems

Humeral (lymphatic) immune system

● B lymphocytes (B-cells) and T lymphocytes (T-cells)

Each B-cell and T-cell is specific for a particular antigen. What this means is that each is able to bind to a particular molecular structure. This response is carried out by antibodies, which are also known as immunoglobulins. These comes in different types: IgG is the most common, followed by IgM, IgA (in mucus) and IgE (in the inflammatory response). These are made of molecules of protein that derive from B-lymphocytes. They circulate in the body fluids (hence humeral: from the old concept of humours) and are transported by the lymphatic system and stored in the lymph nodes. Blood plasma contains 15 different proteins collectively known as complement (see above). These are activated by immunoglobulins, and when activated the complement proteins interact with the humeral immune response.

● B-cells

Antibodies: The humeral antibody system produces antibodies that bind to antigens and identify the antigen complex for destruction (lyse). Antibodies act on antigens in serum and lymph. B-cell antibodies may either be attached to B-cell membranes or free floating in the serum and lymph. The plasma cells live for only 4–5 days but can be reproduced at a rate of 2,000 antibody molecules per second.

Although the general structure of an antibody is similar, a small region at the tip is variable (hypervariable region). Each of these variants binds to a different target (antigen). The unique part of the antigen recognised by the antibody is called an epitope; these epitopes bind with their antibodies and tag them for attack and destruction. See Table 5.8, which shows you how antibodies work.

Table 5.8   How antibodies work

Antibodies produced in the lymph nodes link antigens together causing agglutination (clumping together) of pathogens
Precipitation of antibody molecules that react with soluble antigens (complement)
Activates systems that cause lysis of pathogens (T-cells)
Opsonise (coats) pathogens: identifying them as foreign cells to phagocytes

● T-cells or the mediated system

T-cells are so called because they migrate to the thymus gland to mature. Immunity is given by specific activated T-lymphocytes which destroy (lyse) infected cells, cancerous cells or foreign cells (such as those in transplanted organs). These can be helper, cytotoxic (killer), suppressor or memory T-cells. The mediated system acts on antigens appearing on the surface of individual cells. T-cells produce T-cell receptors, which recognise specific antigens bound to the antigen-presenting structures on the surface of the cell. When a T-cell is presented with an antigen, its receptor binds to the antigen and it is stimulated to divide and reproduce. Killer T-cells (cytotoxic) only recognise antigens coupled to Class I MHC molecules (MHC = major histocompatibility complex). Helper T-cells produce a growth factor called an interleukin, this proliferates the killer T-cells.

Killer T-cells are activated when their T-cell receptor (TCR) binds to this specific antigen in a complex with the MHC Class I receptor of another cell. Recognition of this MHC–antigen complex is aided by a co-receptor on the T-cell called CD8. The T-cell then travels throughout the body in search of cells where the MHC I receptors bear this antigen. When an activated T-cell contacts such cells, it releases cytotoxins, such as perforin, which form pores in the target cell's plasma membrane, allowing ions, water and toxins to enter. T-cell activation is tightly controlled and generally requires a very strong MHC–antigen activation signal, or additional activation signals provided by the helper T-cells. Helper T-cells have no cytotoxic activity and do not kill infected cells or pathogens directly. They instead control the immune response by directing other cells to perform these tasks.

- Natural killer lymphocytes

These are similar to killer cells as they break down target cells but they do not need to interact with other lymphocytes or antibodies.

- Suppressor T-cells

These regulate the overall response of the killer cells and B-cells. They protect uninfected cells and act as a restraining influence when the response is no longer required

Memory cells: the secondary immune response

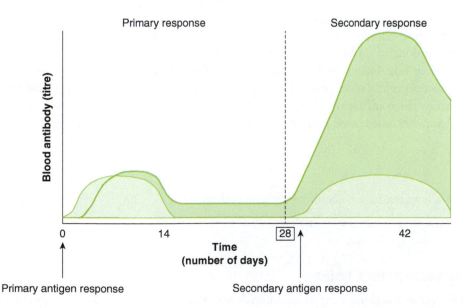

Figure 5.32   Secondary immune response

Memory cells are a part of the acquired immunity system; once the body has been exposed to a disease and survived, a large group of B-cells and T-cells (memory cells) remains capable of producing a secondary immune response should the pathogen reappear in the body. This is called naturally acquired immunity. A secondary immune response is more powerful than the primary response, producing antibodies so quickly that the disease never gets a chance to develop (see Figure 5.32).

The characteristics of the immune systems are summarised in Table 5.9.

Table 5.9   Summary of the immune systems

Innate immune system	Adaptive immune system
Response is non-specific	Pathogen and antigen-specific response
Exposure leads to immediate response	Delay between exposure and response
Cell-mediated and humoral components	Cell-mediated and humoral components
No immunological memory	Immunological memory

When it all goes wrong

When the immune system is functioning normally, it distinguishes 'self' from 'non-self' but sometimes the immune system mistakes its own cells for pathogens, resulting in an autoimmune disease. The immune system attacks the tissue of the body, such as in multiple sclerosis which results from the destruction of myelin sheath of nerve fibres.

The effects of ageing on the immune system (immunosenescence)

The immune system becomes less able to distinguish self from non-self (see above). Therefore, autoimmune disorders become more common (such as arthritis). There are fewer white cells and macrophage and T-cell function slows. This impacts on complement production, which explains why cancer is more common in older people and why they take longer to heal or recover from infection. As the amount of antibody production is less, older people become more susceptible to infections and have trouble fighting them off (reinfection) so that colds and influenza develop into pneumonia. Vaccines become less effective and need to be repeated (boosted) annually.

Go Further 5.10

You can read more about the immune system at:

www.wiley-vch.de/books/sample/3527324127_c01.pdf

The musculoskeletal system

This system is about how locomotion is achieved through muscles moving the skeleton. Muscle tissue is comprised of long filaments (muscle cells) bundled together to

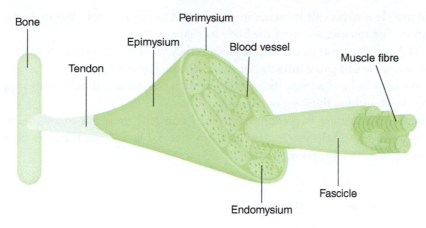

Figure 5.33   Muscle fibre

form muscle fibres (see Figure 5.33), which are also bundled together to form muscles. Muscles attach to the skeleton and this allows movement. The body has approximately 640 different skeletal muscles and most of them are bilateral (found on both sides of the body) and they comprise half of the body weight.

Skeletal muscles are voluntary (unlike cardiac or smooth muscle which is involuntary), and have three main properties:

- Extensibility: ability to change length to lever bones
- Elasticity: ability to return to resting length after being stretched
- Contractility: ability to shorten to produce force

A single elongated cylindrical muscle cell is multinucleated (more than one nucleus). The cell's membrane is called the sarcolemma and its cytoplasm is called sarcoplasm. It contains contractile units called myofibrils made up of actin and myosin in repeated units called sarcomeres (see Figure 5.34) (for more detail, research 'sliding filament theory'). Each cell is coated in a connective tissue called the endomysium and a bundle of cells is collectively known as a fascicle. A bundle of fascicles is surrounded by the perimysium and the whole muscle is surrounded by the epimysium. The function of

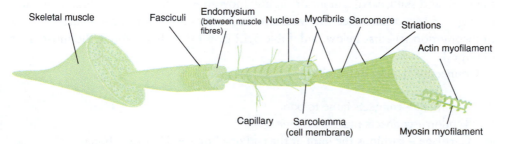

Figure 5.34   Muscle fibre showing sarcomere and myofilament

skeletal muscle is to provide movement, give support to posture and a by-product is heat generation. The muscles also give the body its shape.

Skeletal muscles are antagonistic, this means they work in opposition to one another: when one muscle of a pair contracts, the other relaxes. For example, when one muscle in a pair contracts to bend a joint, its counterpart then contracts and pulls in the opposite direction to straighten the joint out again.

Muscle nomenclature is predominantly in Latin and there are many mnemonics (quite often rude) to help you remember them. See Table 5.10 for the rules on which the naming of muscles is predicated.

Table 5.10   The naming convention for muscles

Location (e.g., the temporalis muscle overlies the temporal bone)

Shape (e.g., the deltoid muscle group is roughly triangular or deltoid shape)

Size (minimus means small, maximus means large, brevis means short and longus means long)

Direction (rectus refers to straight, transverse or oblique means that they run on an angle)

Number of origins (biceps (2), triceps (3), quadriceps (4))

Location of origin and/or insertion (e.g., the sternocleidomastoid is named because it attaches to the sternum and the clavicle and it inserts to the mastoid process of the temporal bone)

The skeletal system

The bony framework of the body (see Figure 5.35) comprises of 206 bones (more in an infant). Its functions are complex and diverse: support, protection, movement, mineral storage and blood cell production. The naming system for bones is given in Figure 5.36 and a mnemonic in Table 5.11.

Bones are primarily made of calcium and collagen, and osteocytes are the long-lived star-shaped cells that make up bone tissue. Osteocytes do not divide but use a complex mechanism involving osteoblasts for reproduction (see Figure 5.37).

Joints

Joints are where bones meet and there are three types: fibrous or immovable, such as the teeth and skull; cartilaginous or slightly moveable, such as the vertebral bones and rib cage; and synovial or freely moveable joints, such as in the limbs and which are used in locomotion (the list below and Table 5.12 give more detail about the movement of bones).

Connective tissues: Remember …

- Ligament – connects bone to bone
- Tendon – connects muscle to bone
- Cartilage – cushions the joint at the end of a bone and between bones
- Bursa – fluid-filled sac that allows bones to move easily over others

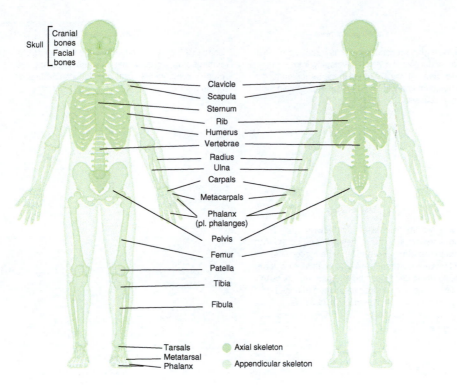

Skull { Cranial bones / Facial bones

Clavicle
Scapula
Sternum
Rib
Humerus
Vertebrae
Radius
Ulna
Carpals
Metacarpals
Phalanx (pl. phalanges)
Pelvis
Femur
Patella
Tibia
Fibula

Tarsals
Metatarsal
Phalanx

● Axial skeleton
○ Appendicular skeleton

Figure 5.35   The skeleton

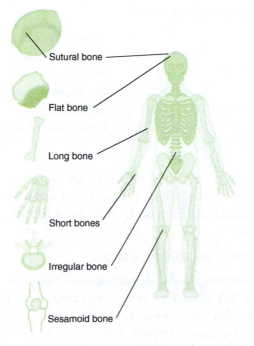

Sutural bone

Flat bone

Long bone

Short bones

Irregular bone

Sesamoid bone

Figure 5.36   The naming convention for bones

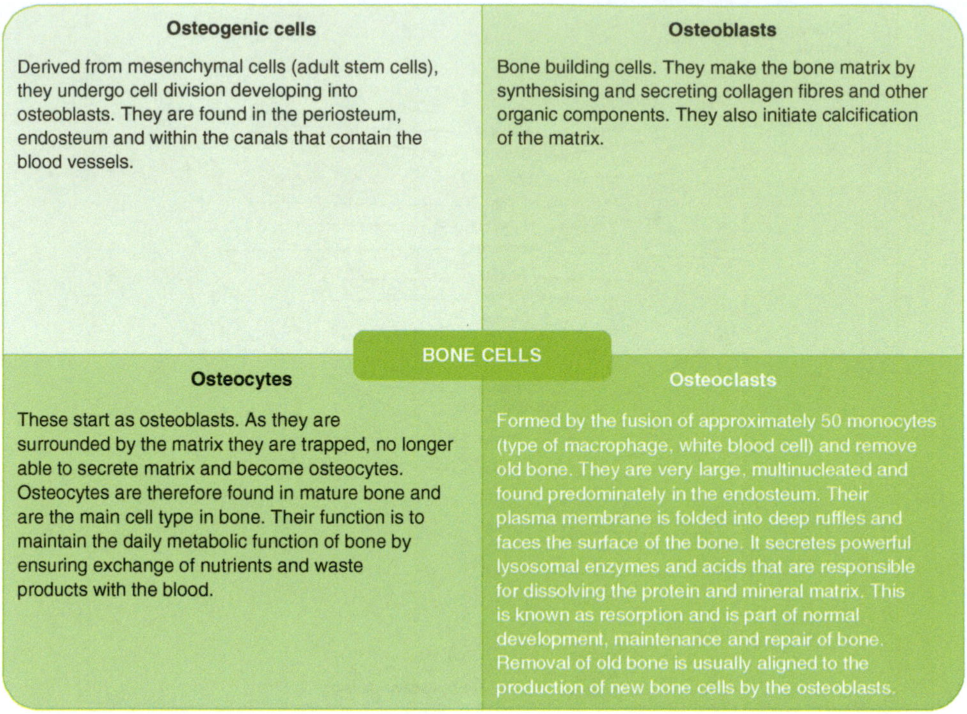

Osteogenic cells	Osteoblasts
Derived from mesenchymal cells (adult stem cells), they undergo cell division developing into osteoblasts. They are found in the periosteum, endosteum and within the canals that contain the blood vessels.	Bone building cells. They make the bone matrix by synthesising and secreting collagen fibres and other organic components. They also initiate calcification of the matrix.

BONE CELLS

Osteocytes	Osteoclasts
These start as osteoblasts. As they are surrounded by the matrix they are trapped, no longer able to secrete matrix and become osteocytes. Osteocytes are therefore found in mature bone and are the main cell type in bone. Their function is to maintain the daily metabolic function of bone by ensuring exchange of nutrients and waste products with the blood.	Formed by the fusion of approximately 50 monocytes (type of macrophage, white blood cell) and remove old bone. They are very large, multinucleated and found predominately in the endosteum. Their plasma membrane is folded into deep ruffles and faces the surface of the bone. It secretes powerful lysosomal enzymes and acids that are responsible for dissolving the protein and mineral matrix. This is known as resorption and is part of normal development, maintenance and repair of bone. Removal of old bone is usually aligned to the production of new bone cells by the osteoblasts.

Figure 5.37 Development of bone cells

Table 5.11 The mnemonic for naming bones: FISSSL

F = Flat	Scapula, sternum, pelvis, ribs
I = Irregular	Vertebrae, facial bones
S = Sutural	Skull bones
S = Short	Carpals and tarsals
S = Sesamoid	Patella
L = Long	Femur, tibia, fibula, humerus, radius and ulnar

Synovial joints (see Figure 5.38) allow different types of movement: **abduction** = the joint moving away from the middle of the body, and **adduction** = the joint moving towards the middle of the body. Both occur at the wrist, shoulder and hip.

The effects of ageing on the musculoskeletal system

Bones stop growing towards the end of adolescence. Nutrition has an impact on the strength of bones as a lack of calcium, protein and other nutrients during growth and development can cause bones to be small. Bones need vitamin D, which is necessary for absorption of calcium from the intestines, and vitamin C, which is necessary for collagen synthesis by osteoblasts. Levels of calcium in the blood depend upon movement

Table 5.12   Synovial joint movements

Joint	Movement
Ball and socket (shoulder/hips)	Wide range of movements
Hinge (ankle/elbow)	Movement is restricted to bending and straightening only
Pivot (atlas – axis, radio – ulnar)	Movement is restricted to one bone rotating about its longitudinal axis
Condyloid (wrist/knuckles)	Allows almost as much movement as the ball and socket
Gliding (fingers/toes)	Allows a limited range of movement in all directions
Saddle (thumb)	The concave area of one bone articulates with the convex area of the adjacent bone and vice versa
Apophyseal (vertebrae)	Hinge-like joints that allow the flexion, extension and torsion of the spine

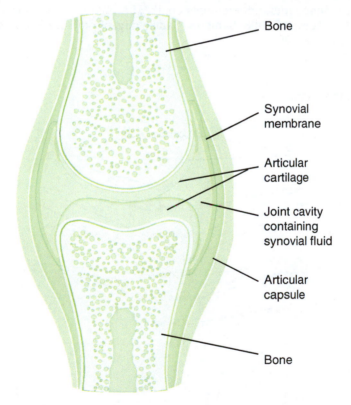

Bone

Synovial membrane

Articular cartilage

Joint cavity containing synovial fluid

Articular capsule

Bone

Figure 5.38   A synovial joint

of calcium into or out of bone. This is controlled by two hormones: the parathyroid hormone increases it and calcitonin lowers it.

As we age, bone matrix production falls leading to bone loss, collagen production also falls leading to brittle bones, and for women, the rate of bone loss increases 10-fold after menopause. This leads to increased risk of fractures and can cause deformity (such as 'Dowager's hump'), loss of height (approximately 2 inches by age 80 caused by compression of vertebrae), pain, stiffness and loosening teeth.

As we age our muscles generally decrease in strength, endurance, size and weight. The muscular system ages due to loss of muscle density, lack of movement due to pain, and slower muscle–nerve interaction due to a poorer response to stimuli. Typically, we lose about 23% of our muscle mass by age 80 as both the number and size of muscle fibres decrease. These changes may be more the result of inactivity, poor nutrition and chronic illness or disease rather than the result of ageing per se and much of this decrease in muscle mass can be prevented by maintaining physical fitness.

Go Further 5.11

You can read more on the skeletal and muscular system at:

www.pearsonschoolsandfecolleges.co.uk/FEAndVocational/SportsStudies/
ALevel/OCRALevelPE2008/Samples/SamplepagesfromOCRASPEStudentBook/
chapter1_sample.pdf

The endocrine system

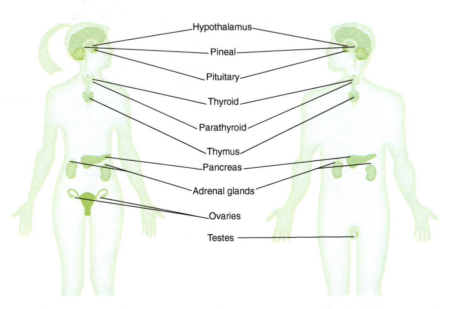

Figure 5.39   The endocrine system

This system is the collection of glands that produce the hormones that regulate metabolism, growth and development, tissue function, sexual function and reproduction. The glands are: the hypothalamus, pineal gland, thymus, thyroid gland, parathyroid glands, pituitary gland, adrenal glands, pancreas, ovaries (in females) and testes (in males). Hormones circulate through the body and target their associated organs and tissues.

Imbalances within the system can lead to infertility, thyroid ailments (hyper/hypothy-roidism) and in the case of the pancreas, diabetes.

Go Further 5. 12

You can read more on the endocrine system at:

www.lamission.edu/lifesciences/lecturenote/AliPhysio1/Endrocrine%20System.pdf

---

Wound healing

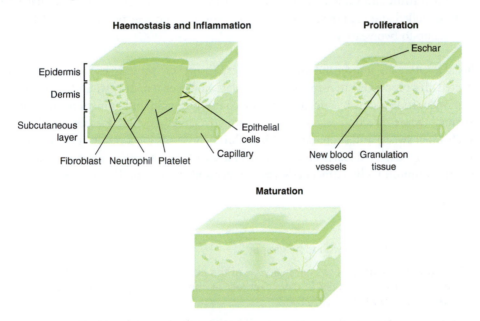

Figure 5.40   Wound healing

Wound healing happens in three stages:

[1] **Inflammation**, where pyrogens begin the process of killing invaders (see the immune system above) causing swelling, pain, heat and redness. In response to damage, the blood vessels constrict (haemostasis) and seal as the platelets are trapped in nets of fibrinogen which form a clot and stop bleeding. Bacteria and debris are phagocytosed and removed, which is characterised by the infiltration of neutrophils, macrophages and lymphocytes.

[2] **Proliferation** as the wound begins to grow new healthy granulation tissue along the wound bed. Angiogenesis is the process of growing new blood vessels within tissues made of extracellular matrix and collagen. Epithelial cells crawl across wound bed to cover it, the wound then contracts and closes (see Figure 5.41).

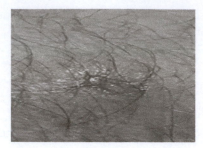

Figure 5.41   A healing burn

[3] **Maturation** and remodelling occurs after the wound has healed over. Collagen is remodelled and realigned, dermal tissue is formed and scar tissue reduces (this can take up to two years).

This describes an uneventful healing process, however, sometimes wounds become infected, this process is interrupted or incomplete, and even a mature wound can suddenly burst open. Indications of infection include continuing pain, inflammation, an unpleasant smell (some infectious agents have a distinctive smell, such as *Pseudomonas* bacteria which smell sweet) and suppuration. Most chronic wounds are a result of ischemia, vascular incompetence, diabetes and decubitus ulcers. Other factors in delayed healing are immunocompromise by iatrogenesis, age, gender and (over or under) nutrition.

Go Further 5.13

You can read more on wound healing at:

The wound healing process: an overview of the cellular and molecular mechanisms by T. Velnar, T. Bailey and V. Smrkolj, in the *Journal of International Medical Research*, 2009, 37(5): 1528–42.

http://journals.sagepub.com/doi/abs/10.1177/147323000903700531

CHAPTER SUMMARY

- This chapter has introduced you to basic anatomy and physiology and given details of each system as it ages. The chapter cannot replace a good A&P book and suggestions for further research are given throughout the chapter. You can download *Nurses: Test Yourself Anatomy and Physiology*, also Marieb's in-depth test bank, which are both in the Further Reading below.
- Watch YouTube videos and podcasts to aid your understanding when you feel overwhelmed. I also really recommend drawing diagrams if you are a kinetic learner.
- Wound healing is a specialism in nursing (tissue viability) but it is important to understand the mechanics of both the immune system in action and healing process to support the care of your patients.

📖 FURTHER READING

Websites

Top tip: if you type into your browser the body system you are interested in and put PDF after it, you can will find whole chapters you can download.

- *Fundamentals of Anatomy and Physiology*: www.fundamentalsofanatomy.com/ (for nurses)
- Howard Hughes Medical Institute – Biointeractive: www.hhmi.org/biointeractive
- Inner Body: www.innerbody.com/
- Khan Academy – Human Anatomy and Physiology: www.khanacademy.org/science/health-and-medicine/human-anatomy-and-physiology

Books and articles

- British Pain Society (2014) *Suggested Reading List*. Available at: www.britishpainsociety.org/suggested-reading-list/.
- Guo, S. and DiPietro, L. (2010) Factors affecting wound healing. *Journal of Dental Research*, 89(3): 219–29.
- Marieb, E. (2012) *Essentials of Human Anatomy and Physiology Test Bank* (10th edn). Available at: https://cjbaguhin246.wordpress.com/2013/08/07/marieb-essentials-of-human-anatomy-physiology-10th-test-bank/.
- Marieb, E. and Hoehn, K. (2015) *Human Anatomy & Physiology*. London: Pearson.
- McKissock, C. (2014) *Great Ways to Learn Anatomy and Physiology*. Basingstoke: Palgrave.
- Peate, I. and Nair, M. (2016) *Fundamentals of Anatomy and Physiology: For Nursing and Healthcare Students*. Oxford: Wiley.
- Riley, K. (2014) *Wound Care* (Nursing and Health Survival Guides). Oxford: Routledge.
- Rogers, K. and Scott, W. (2011) *Nurses: Test Yourself Anatomy and Physiology*. Available at: downloadnursingpdf.blogspot.com/2013/02/nurses-test-yourself-in-anatomy.html.
- Tierney, K. (2012) *Anatomy & Physiology Student Workbook: 2,000 Puzzles & Quizzes* (3rd edn). CreateSpace Independent Publishing Platform.
- Waugh, A. and Grant, A. (2014) *Ross and Wilson: Anatomy and Physiology in Health and Illness* (12th edn). London: Elsevier.

6

PREVENTION AND CONTROL OF INFECTION

Deborah Gee

Prevention and management of infection is the responsibility of all staff working in health and social care.

Royal College of Nursing (2012)

This chapter will introduce you to the importance of infection control within health and social care settings. You will understand the core principles in managing the spread of infection through institutions and the preventative measures available. You will also examine the legislation that supports infection control. This chapter links with bioscience, which was the focus of Chapter 5, and will remind you of the body's immune system functions.

Glossary

- **CQC** Care Quality Commission
- **Evidence-based practice** Ways of working that have been proved to be effective
- **Healthcare-Associated Infection (HCAI)** Infection as a result of being in a healthcare setting
- **HSE** The Health and Safety Executive
- **PPE** Personal protective clothing
- **RCN** The Royal College of Nursing
- **RIDDOR** Reporting of Injuries, Diseases and Dangerous Occurrences Regulations 2013

INTRODUCTION

Over the past two decades, individuals working within clinical practice have faced increasing challenges in managing the spread of infection within the healthcare environment. Generally, when a patient acquires an infection following admission to the healthcare setting this is classified as a Healthcare-Associated Infection (HCAI). Recent research by Cassini estimated that between 2011 and 2012, more than 2.5 millionhospital-acquired infections were caught across Europe, leading to 90,000 deaths (Cassini et al., 2016).

HCAIs bring increased morbidity and mortality to the patients. Patients with infection are likely to experience increased pain and discomfort, not forgetting the financial burden prolonged treatments can bring to both the care provider and the patient themselves.

Using an evidence-based approach, this chapter will provide those working in health and social care settings with the knowledge and skills to practise safe infection prevention and control when working with service users. It will also introduce some of the health and safety legislation linked to safety and will offer suggested areas for critical reflection and further reading.

THE IMPORTANCE OF INFECTION CONTROL IN HEALTHCARE PRACTICE

Within healthcare practice over the past two decades there has been a plethora of government initiatives to address the increasing numbers of healthcare associated infections (Figure 6.1).

With the number of infections rising the subsequent extensive use of available antibiotics to treat these infections, has resulted in an increased number of infections such as MRSA (methicillin resistant *Staphylococcus aureus*), VRE (vancomycin-

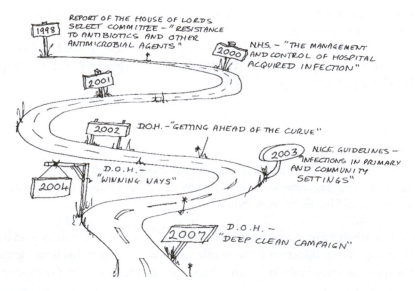

Figure 6.1   Timeline of initiatives

resistant enterococci), C-diff (*Clostridium difficile*, E-coli (*Escherichia coli*) and ESBL (extended-spectrum beta-lactamases), all of which are increasingly resistant to many of the current antibiotics available, and this brings increased challenges for the health and social care profession.

In 2012, the Royal College of Nursing (RCN) provided practitioners with a toolkit with an overarching framework to help meet the challenge of reducing, and sustaining the reduction in healthcare-associated infections (HCAIs). However, the reduction of HCAIs remains high on the government's safety and quality agenda and in the general public's expectations for quality of care. The *Code of Practice on the Prevention and Control of Infections* (Department of Health, 2015) applies to all registered providers of healthcare and adult social care in England. The Code of Practice (Part 2) sets out the ten criteria against which the Care Quality Commission (CQC) will judge a registered provider on how it complies with the infection prevention requirements set out in regulations.

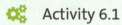 Activity 6.1

Hospitals and care providers for many years have recognised the significance of infection prevention and control and employ specialist infection control staff. Are you able to identify nominated person(s) in your workplace?

CORE PRINCIPLES IN INFECTION PREVENTION AND CONTROL

The prevention and control of infection is the responsibility of all staff working within health and social care settings, and all have a duty to ensure that those they care for are not at risk from poor practice.

The *English National Point Prevalence Survey* reported that in 2011 6.4% of the hospital population developed a HCAI (Health Protection Agency, 2012). The acquisition of a HCAI has potential implications for:

- Patients
- Visitors
- Staff
- Workers such as electricians and plumbers working in buildings
- The employing organisation, e.g. healthcare trust, care home, hospice etc.
- The National Health Service (NHS)

The effective implementation of basic core principles is the first step in managing the control and spread of infection because poor practice related to hygiene increases the risk of hospital-acquired infections, and this in turn can lead to pain, distress, unwanted exposure to medication (and negative side effects), lengthened hospital stays, long-term complications and even death for your patient. We must also consider the impact upon the NHS and other healthcare providers of such things as increased costs, reduced public confidence and reduced staff morale.

The core principles of infection prevention and control are:

- Effective hand washing
- Protective clothing
- Barrier or isolation nursing
- Laundry and waste management
- Cleanliness of the environment
- Decontamination of equipment

 Activity 6.2

Consider what the potential implications are when a service user has acquired a HCAI.

Hand hygiene

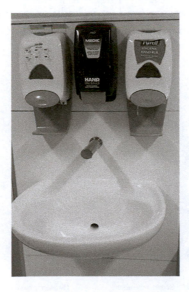

Figure 6.2   Hand hygiene

One of the most effective and non-invasive ways of preventing HCAIs is through good hand hygiene (see Figure 6.2). Hands carry two different types of micro-organisms: transient and resident. Infection can occur when micro-organisms are transferred from one patient to another, either from equipment or the environment to patients or between the staff with a disruption to a patient's 'normal bacterial flora', potentially resulting in infection.

Transient micro-organisms are found on the skin surface. These are readily acquired from contact with other body sites, people and the environment, and are easily transferred to others. The disruption to the normal body flora can predispose the individual to infection if the bacteria are being transferred from one part of the body where they are not normally resident. For example, if faecal bacteria from the groin is transferred to the face during washing, or performing mouth care without the healthcare worker undertaking effective hand hygiene or changing their gloves.

Resident micro-organisms are part of our normal skin flora and are found in deeper skin layers, hair follicles and sweat glands and they are more difficult to remove than transient micro-organisms.

It is essential for all healthcare workers to ensure they clean their hands at the right times and in the right way.

How should we wash our hands?

Despite awareness of the importance of effective hand washing, studies repeatedly show that effective hand washing is dependent upon many factors including the selection of the appropriate cleansing product in addition to the technique used (WHO, 2009). Figure 6.3 shows commonly missed areas as a result of poor technique.

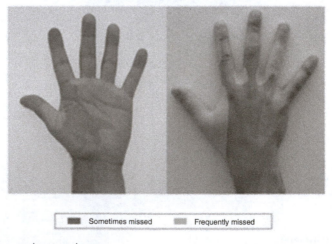

Sometimes missed   Frequently missed

Figure 6.3   Commonly missed areas

In practice, there are generally three different ways hands are cleaned:

[1] Soap and water – effective in removing dirt and soiling and transient micro-organisms.
[2] Antimicrobial detergent – effective in removing dirt and soiling and more effective in removing resident micro-organisms.
[3] Alcohol-based hand rubs – effective on non-soiled hands, quick and effective way of destroying transient bacteria. Note: not effective with *Clostridium difficile* infections (WHO, 2009).

What is the correct technique? Effective hand washing involves three stages: *preparation*, *washing* and *rinsing*, and *drying*.

- **Preparation**: Wet hands under tepid running water before applying the recommended amount of liquid soap or an antimicrobial preparation.
- **Washing**: Hands should be washed and rinsed thoroughly. The hand wash solution must come into contact with all of the surfaces of the hand and the hands should be rubbed together for 10–15 seconds (EPIC 3, Loveday, 2014).

Within healthcare practice the consensus across the literature would appear to be that the six-step approach first provided by Ayliffe et al. in the late 1970s is the most effective method (see Figure 6.4):

[1] Rub hands palm to palm.
[2] Rub right palm over the back of the other hand with interlaced fingers and vice versa.
[3] Rub palm to palm with the fingers interlaced.
[4] Rub the backs of fingers to opposing palms with fingers interlocked.
[5] Use rotational rubbing of the left thumb clasped in the right palm and vice versa.
[6] Use rotational rubbing, backwards and forwards with clasped fingers of the right hand in the left palm and vice versa. (Ayliffe et al., 1978)

- **Drying**: In healthcare practice always use good-quality paper towels to dry the hands thoroughly (EPIC 3, Loveday, 2014).

Go Further 6.1

You might read the original research by Aycliffe, Babb and Quoraishi. You can find it here: http://jcp.bmj.com/content/jclinpath/31/10/923.full.pdf. It is an interesting read, as due to poor hand washing, several research participants became very unwell.

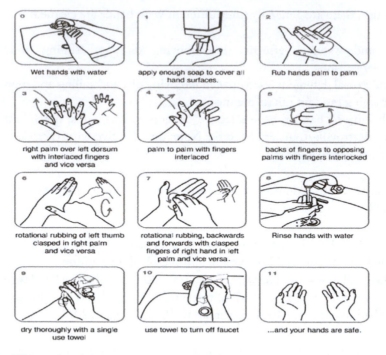

Figure 6.4   Effective hand cleaning

Activity 6.3

Explore some of the current literature from the World Health Organization (WHO.org). Consider the current recommendations and some of the health education campaigns to promote effective handwashing. Can you recall seeing any of these health education messages in your clinical areas?

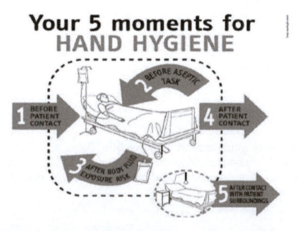

Figure 6.5   Hand hygiene at the point of care

The World Health Organization (WHO, 2006) advocates five key moments for hand hygiene (see Figure 6.5):

[1] **Before patient contact:** The need to decontaminate our hands prior to contact with a patient and this includes arrival on duty.

[2] **Before aseptic task:** The aseptic technique is used in practice to reduce the risk of infection occurring as a result of a procedure taking place. This usually follows a set of specific actions. Staff expected to perform aseptic procedures will receive appropriate training and will be deemed as competent before performing this independently. Practice examples where the need for aseptic technique is required are when changing a patient's wound dressings or when dealing with intravenous fluid administration.

[3] **After body fluid exposure risk:** Such as blood, faeces, vomit and urine. This includes after protective gloves have been removed as it is important to consider that:

- gloves may become damaged in use (the damage may be visible or microscopic)
- hands may also be contaminated accidentally when gloves are being removed
- the environment inside the glove may promote microbial growth on the user's hands
- hand washing after taking off gloves may also remove particles of the material that the gloves are made of, e.g. latex, and so reduce the risk of developing an allergy.

[4] **After patient contact:** For example, when undertaking moving and handling tasks.

[5] **After contact with patient surroundings:** As micro-organisms live on both hard surfaces and soft furnishings (Figure 6.6).

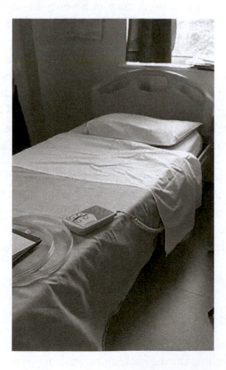

Figure 6.6   Ward bed

Personal protective equipment

When working in the health or social care setting, health and safety regulations (HSE, 1992) state that in order to protect you from any risk to your health and safety your employer must undertake appropriate risk assessments and provide you with the personal protective equipment (PPE) necessary to reduce the risks. All employees must be provided with information, instruction and training on the PPE available for use.

Some of the most common pieces of PPE are: disposable gloves, disposable plastic aprons, and masks, visors and eye protection.

Disposable gloves

These are essential in the prevention and control of infection within healthcare practice. However, it is important to wear gloves only when necessary as unnecessary use can arguably undermine the current hand hygiene initiatives. There is also the potential health risk to the healthcare worker, as wearing gloves when they are not necessary can lead to other problems such as contact dermatitis or exacerbation of other skin problems.

There are many different types of disposable gloves available to choose from and health workers need to ensure that they use the correct gloves and the that the ones chosen are fit for purpose.

Powdered latex and natural rubber latex gloves should not generally be used as they increase the risk of allergic reaction in patients and staff with existing allergies. Latex can also lead to allergic contact dermatitis and occupational asthma in sensitised individuals. If latex gloves are to be used, they must only be used following a thorough risk assessment for suitability and safety. If they are selected for use they must be low protein and single use (HSE, 2011).

In addition to the latex, other chemicals known as accelerators can present a risk of work-related dermatitis. The Health and Safety Executive states that health surveillance checks should be carried out on those exposed to hazardous substances.

Under the Reporting of Injuries, Diseases and Dangerous Occurrences Regulations (RIDDOR, 2013) there is a legal requirement to report occupational asthma or dermatitis related to normal rubber latex to the Health and Safety Executive (HSE).

[1] Neoprene and nitrile gloves are good alternatives to natural rubber latex. These are a synthetic glove and have been shown in clinical studies to be comparable in use to the rubber latex ones.

[2] Vinyl gloves can be used for many tasks in the healthcare setting but may not be appropriate when handling bloodstained products, cytotoxic drugs or other high risk substances.

[3] Polythene gloves are not suitable for use in healthcare practice.

Disposable plastic aprons

These provide a physical barrier between clothing/skin and prevent contamination and wetting of uniforms/clothing during bathing or washing or equipment cleaning.

Aprons should be worn whenever there is a risk of contamination with blood or bodily fluids and when the patient has a suspected or known infection.

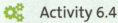

Activity 6.4

Employers provide different coloured plastic aprons for use in the clinical area – how many can you identify in your area? What is the rationale for this?

Masks, visors and eye protection

These items should be worn when it is likely that blood or bodily fluids may splash into the eyes, face or mouth. They should be worn when there is likelihood of exposure to bodily fluids, such as in childbirth, trauma or operation theatre environments.

Masks may also be necessary if infection may be spread by an airborne route. All staff should be trained in how to fit a mask safely. If we are at risk in our environment, then the employer has a legal obligation to provide this protection under the Health and Safety at Work Act 1974 (Section 9).

Barrier or isolation nursing

Within healthcare practice, there are times when patients need to be barrier nursed or cared for in isolation. This is sometimes necessary to reduce the risk of spreading infection, including those resistant to antibiotic treatment, and to protect patients who are more susceptible to infection, for example those who may have a compromised immune system because of their illness or the medications they are taking.

Barrier nursing involves the healthcare practitioner taking extra precautions to prevent the spread of the germs. Isolation nursing usually involves the patient being in a side room. The infection prevention control professional from your practice area will be able to offer specific advice regarding this.

Safe handling and disposal of waste

Any healthcare worker who produces waste as a part of their job is classified as a 'waste producer' (RCN, 2012). Within health and social care practice waste is produced from those providing health and social care to patients, either in their own homes or within a healthcare organisation. There are three categories of waste: clinical, hazardous and offensive (Royal College of Nursing, 2014).

Waste reduction, segregation and disposal are all crucial to sustaining a healthy environment and reducing costs. As healthcare waste can include human waste and bodily fluids in addition to sharps (needles, scalpels, glass vials etc.) and other biohazardous materials that may be infectious, it is essential that all waste products are disposed of correctly.

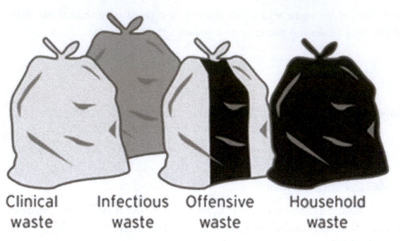

| Clinical waste | Infectious waste | Offensive waste | Household waste |

Figure 6.7   Waste bags

All health and social care organisations should have their own policy which will specify how an organisation manages its waste and identifies who is responsible for this within the organisation. This policy should provide employees with guidance and procedures to ensure that they dispose of waste safely and in compliance with all relevant legislation (Department of Health, 2013a, 2013b).

Activity 6.5

As an employee working within health and social care practice, you should be aware of your organisation's policy and understand how it impacts on your everyday activities. Take a few moments to reflect on this. If you are not aware of the waste policy, or do not understand how it affects you, ask your line manager.

The safe disposal of waste from health and social care is dependent upon the healthcare worker being able to classify the category of waste and use the correct waste container. The RCN (2014) highlight that effective segregation is not only essential for compliance with waste regulations, it is essential to promote good health and safety at work. The *Health Care Waste Management Manual* (DH, 2013b) suggests use of an appropriate classification framework to support healthcare workers in this process. The RCN (2014) also provide further information on how to appropriately classify waste and points out that 'This may be a bag for soft wastes or more rigid container for sharps or medicinal wastes'.

The *Health Care Waste Management Manual* (Department of Health, 2013b, Section 3.2) provides suggested colours for waste containers which can be used to quickly identify the types of waste that should be disposed of within them.

Colour coding for waste containers is important as it makes clear the end disposal/treatment route of the waste.

Whichever colour is used, the waste producer is subject to their duty of care (a legal requirement), and should ensure any container is clearly labelled in a manner that makes the subsequent holder aware of its contents.

Safe handling of sharps

Sharps are items (or parts of items) that could cause cuts or puncture wounds, including needles, the needle part of a syringe, scalpel and other blades, broken glass ampoules and the patient end of an infusion set (cannula/Venflon etc.).

The use of sharps within a procedure can increase the risk of injuries, and therefore to ensure that those working with sharps reduce their risk of injury and infection it is essential that sharps are used and disposed of appropriately (Health and Safety at Work Act 1974).

In May 2013, the European Sharps Directive came into force in the UK. This states that the use of sharps should be eliminated where possible, and employers should consider the use of safety engineered sharps devices where elimination is not possible.

Table 6.1 summarises sharps best practice.

Cleanliness of the environment

All care providers must make sure that the care they provide is safe for service users. They must ensure that they take appropriate measures to prevent and control the spread

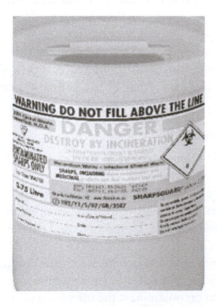

Figure 6.8   Sharps box

Table 6.1   Sharps best practice points

Ensure syringes and needles are placed as complete items straight into a sharps container (see Figure 6.8) following use

Needles should never be re-sheathed or re-capped

All sharps containers should conform to UN standard 3291 and British Standard 7320

Sharps containers should not be overfilled

Staff should attend training on the safe use of sharps, including safety engineered devices

Staff should report sharps injuries in line with local reporting procedures

---

Source: *Essential Practice for Infection Prevention and Control* (RCN, 2012)

of infection, ensuring that the premises and any equipment used are safe, and where applicable available in sufficient quantities (Department of Health, 2015).

A dirty clinical environment is one of the factors that may contribute towards infection rates. Effective cleaning to remove contaminants such as dust, faeces, blood and bodily fluids will help reduce the risk of cross-infection.

There are several different methods for cleaning: traditional methods such as detergent with water and microfibre cloths, the use of appropriate cleaning wipes for some items, and the specialist technologies such as hydrogen peroxide vapour cleaning (RCN, 2012).

Local policies should be consulted with regards to the cleaning regime and all healthcare workers have a duty to ensure that standards of cleanliness are maintained, reporting any concerns as per employer policy.

Spillages of all blood and bodily fluids should be dealt with quickly following your workplace written policy for managing these incidents. You should understand these *before* such incidents happen.

This policy should include details of the chemicals staff should use to deal with the incident properly, for example there will be differences if the spillage is on a hard surface or a carpeted floor either in a care setting or in a patient's home.

Decontamination of equipment

Within healthcare practice there are several specific types of equipment available for use (see Table 6.2).

Decontamination of equipment is a term used for the removal of microbial contamination to make an item safe. All multi-patient use equipment needs to be cleaned and decontaminated in between patients. The process can involve cleaning, disinfection and sterilisation.

Cleaning is the most effective way of reducing the risk of infection from equipment, and is essential in the process of disinfection and sterilisation.

Disinfection is used to decontaminate the micro-organisms from the environment, and multi-use equipment such as beds, commodes, bath chairs and blood pressure cuffs.

Table 6.2   Permissible use of different types of equipment

Type of equipment	Used more than once?	Examples
Single use	No	Needles, syringes, thermometer covers
Single patient use	Yes, for the same patient but still needs to be cleaned in between use	Pulse oximeter probes, nebulisers
Re-useable multi-patient use	Yes, but needs decontamination in between use	Beds, commodes, shower chairs, blood pressure cuffs

Sterilisation is the process involving the removal of all types of micro-organisms, however it is impossible to ensure that every micro-organism is destroyed, and therefore effective thorough cleaning is essential in the process to optimise the results.

All health and social care staff must be aware of the implications of ineffective decontamination of equipment, and employing organisations need to ensure that all staff are trained and competent to ensure they keep themselves and patients/service users safe.

THE BODY'S DEFENCE SYSTEMS

Individuals in healthcare settings such as hospitals are vulnerable to the risk of infection for several reasons, including their reduced immunity, the presence of invasive devices and the fact that they have increased risk of being in contact with other patients who are suffering from infection.

Infections themselves are generally caused by micro-organisms and the term 'infectious agent' is frequently used to describe these. The body, however, has its own natural defences and has several specific ways of protecting itself from infection. (You can find more discussion of the immune system in Chapter 5, Bioscience.)

The body's defence mechanisms are divided into two categories: non-specific defence mechanisms and specific defence mechansims. Let's look at non-specific mechanisms first. These are effective against any invader.

Non-specific defence

The skin protects most of the body surface, but there are also other protective features, for example, **sticky mucus**, which traps microbes and other foreign materials and prevents tissues from drying out, and **body fluids** that can contain antimicrobial substances, for example, gastric juices contain hydrochloric acids. Saliva, which washes the surface of the teeth, also contains lysosomes and enzymes that can break down bacteria. These are classed as the first lines of non-specific defence. They prevent entry and minimise further passage of microbes and other foreign material into the body.

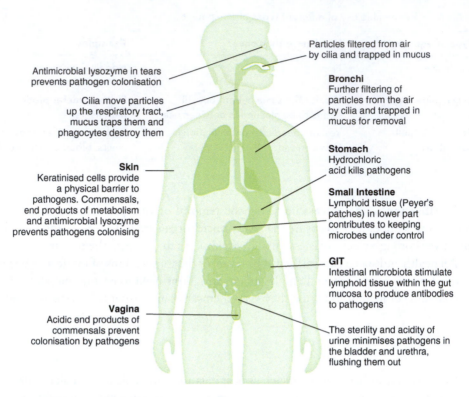

Antimicrobial lysozyme in tears
prevents pathogen colonisation

Cilia move particles
up the respiratory tract,
mucus traps them and
phagocytes destroy them

Skin
Keratinised cells provide
a physical barrier to
pathogens. Commensals,
end products of metabolism
and antimicrobial lysozyme
prevents pathogens colonising

Vagina
Acidic end products of
commensals prevent
colonisation by pathogens

Particles filtered from air
by cilia and trapped in mucus

Bronchi
Further filtering of
particles from the air
by cilia and trapped in
mucus for removal

Stomach
Hydrochloric
acid kills pathogens

Small Intestine
Lymphoid tissue (Peyer's
patches) in lower part
contributes to keeping
microbes under control

GIT
Intestinal microbiota stimulate
lymphoid tissue within the gut
mucosa to produce antibodies
to pathogens

The sterility and acidity of
urine minimises pathogens in
the bladder and urethra,
flushing them out

Figure 6.9   Non-specific defence

Healthy, intact skin and mucus membrane provide an effective barrier. The sebum and sweat excreted provide a good defence to pathogens as they both contain antibacterial and antifungal substances. Epithelial membranes lining body cavities like the respiratory, urinary and digestive tracts, although delicate, are also well defended by

Table 6.3   Natural antimicrobial substances

Hydrochloric acid	Kills most ingested microbes
Lysozyme	Antibacterial enzyme. Destroys bacterial cell walls but does not affect viruses or other pathogens. Found in tears but not in other body secretions like sweat, urine or cerebrospinal fluid
Antibodies	Protective proteins found coating membranes and body fluids and inactive bacteria
Saliva	Secreted into mouth and washes away debris, preventing bacteria and tooth decay
Interferons	Chemicals produced by T-lymphocytes and macrophages. They prevent viral replication in cells
Complement	System of approximately 20 proteins found in blood and tissues (see also Chapter 5)

antibacterial secretions. The epithelia produce more secretions, often acidic, containing antibodies and enzymes as well as sticky mucus for trapping passing microbes. Table 6.3 lists natural antimicrobial substances.

Another of the non-specific defence mechanisms is **phagocytosis**. This is known as 'cell eating'. The phagocytic defence cells such as macrophages and neutrophils are the body's first line of cellular defence. These cells naturally migrate to the site of inflammation and infection and engulf the targets. They indiscriminately digest and destroy foreign cells.

The **inflammatory response** is the physical response to tissue damage. Its purpose is protective: to isolate, inactivate and remove both the cause and the damaged tissues.

Another defence mechanism is **immunological surveillance.** A population of lymphocytes called NK (natural killer) cells patrol the body looking for abnormal cells. Once a cell is detected the NK cells destroy it.

Specific defence

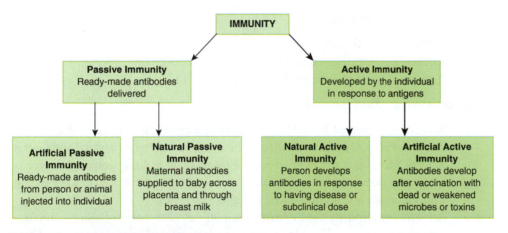

Figure 6.10   Specific defence

Specific defence is when the body generates a specific response against any substance it identifies as foreign. These substances are known as *antigens* and include:

- pollen from flowers and plants
- bacteria and other microbes
- cancer cells or transplanted tissue cells.

These antigens then induce the immune system to produce antibodies and a specific immune response (see Figure 6.10).

If the body's first line of non-specific defences is overwhelmed, then there is an activation of the powerful immune system. Immunity has three key attributes:

[1] Specificity – immune response directed at a specific antigen.

[2] Memory – the response usually forms a memory and therefore if the body is faced with the same challenge again, it will act faster.

[3] Tolerance – the cells of the immune system can be aggressive and destructive. Healthy 'self' cells display marker proteins that tell the immune cells that they are 'OK'. Issues can happen when 'non-self' cells are present, such as transplanted cells and cancer cells.

Types of immunity

[1] Cellular immunity

- Carried out by T-cells. When the T-cell encounters an antigen for the first time, it becomes sensitised to it.
- Antigen-presenting cell (macrophage). Macrophages are like pacman, they chase down and eat (by phagocytosis) invading bacteria, they then mature into antigen-presenting cells to attract T cells and to produce cytokines (antibodies).
- Infected cells are killed by cytotoxic T-cells.

[2] Antibody or humoral immunity

- Carried out by B-cells.
- Antibodies are produced and remain in the bloodstream.
- Antibodies bind to antigens and deactivate them.

[3] Natural and acquired immunity

- Some of the activated T- and B-cells become memory cells. The next time an individual meets up with the same antigen the immune system can respond and destroy it. Depending upon the route of entry into the body and the amount and type of antigen produced, the immunity can be strong or weak, short-lived or long-lasting.
- Immunity can also be influenced by inherited genes.
- An immune response can be sparked not only by infection but also by immunisation with vaccines. Vaccines contain specially treated micro-organisms. Once administered, they provoke an immune response to the specific disease.
- Immunity can also be transferred from one individual to another. The immunological responses of a baby are generally weak, however prior to birth the mother will transfer additional antibodies to the baby to boost its immune system. This protection can be further enhanced by mothers who breastfeed their babies; however this passive immunity typically lasts only a few weeks or months (NHS Choices, 2017).

WHEN INFECTION OCCURS

Despite the body's specific and non-specific defences against infection there are occasions when infections do occur. However, certain conditions need to be met for a micro-organism or infectious disease to be spread from person to person. This process is referred to as the 'chain of infection' (see Figure 6.11).

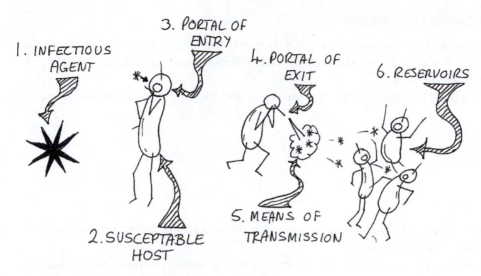

Figure 6.11   The chain of infection

The chain of infection

The infectious agent

Germs (the infectious agent) are generally all around us and play an important part in helping us remain healthy. There are also many germs that are not helpful to our health and can cause disease. The challenge arises when a germ leaves its usual 'healthy' place of residence and travels elsewhere in the body.

The reservoir

This 'place' where germs can live and multiply is called a **reservoir**. This can be a person, who may be either a service user or a member of staff. **BUT** ... it can also be any part of the surrounding area of a health or social care setting, such as fixtures and fittings, including soft furnishings, in addition to any equipment used for patient care.

The portal of exit from the reservoir

The portal of exit can vary depending upon the type of infection. There are both human and non-human means by which the germ can escape.

- **Human –** a healthcare worker touches a used commode, and some of the germs move onto that person's hands. Their hands are now the 'portal of exit' – how the germs are able to move from the commode to another place.
- **Non-human** portals include items of equipment that have not been properly cleaned, such as commodes, bed mattresses, pillows and reusable equipment, which would become the infectious agent (portal of infection).

Modes/means of transmission

Awareness of the methods by which a disease is transmitted is important in infection control; it also highlights the importance of effective hand washing in controlling the spread of infection.

The most common modes of transmission that occur in the care environment are:

- Contact
- Droplet
- Airborne

Contact spread

In contact spread, the susceptible person has either direct or indirect contact with the infected source or reservoir.

Direct (patient) contact occurs when there is actual physical contact between the source and the susceptible person. It is necessary for the source and the susceptible person to be exposed to skin and body secretions via close contact. Remember that organisms can also be transmitted from one part of a person's body, such as their skin, to another part of their own body or to another person, for example, touching a wound.

Indirect (contaminated object) transmission usually occurs when a piece of equipment is used on more than one person and has not been properly cleaned in between uses.

Droplet transmission

Droplet particles cannot be transmitted beyond a radius of a few feet of the source. The large particles generally expelled from respiratory secretions by coughing, sneezing or talking rapidly settle on horizontal surfaces or are deposited on the susceptible person's conjunctivae, nasal membranes or mouth. For instance, viral influenza pathogens are transmitted this way.

Airborne spread

Airborne particles are disseminated having a true airborne phase; this is usually a distance of several feet or more between the source and the susceptible person. Pathogens that are transmitted this way include varicella and tuberculosis.

Portals of entry

Microbes can enter the body through four sites:

- Respiratory tract
- Gastrointestinal tract

- Urogenital tract
- Breaks in the skin surface

The portals of entry in healthcare practice are listed in Table 6.4.

Table 6.4   Portals of entry in healthcare practice

An opening to the skin
Catheter being placed into the bladder (suprapubic or urinary)
Enteral feeding
Central venous catheterisation
Injections/used needles

A susceptible host

The development of an infection from any transferred pathogens is dependent upon the ability of the organism to cause disease and the body's ability to resist it. As we have seen in this chapter, the ability of the body to defend itself is called immunity, and previous exposure and immune response will also play a role. Healthy people are generally able to 'fight off' infection; however some (both apparently well and unwell) people are unable to fight infection, making them susceptible hosts when their bodies are invaded.

Implications for practice: sepsis

Sepsis is a common and potentially life-threatening condition triggered by infection that can lead to shock, organ failure or death. Sepsis claims 44,000 lives annually in the UK (Sepsis Trust, 2017). In 2002, following international collaboration, the Surviving Sepsis Campaign developed the 'Sepsis Six' guidance to support those caring for patients at risk of sepsis. The campaign has continued worldwide with the commitment to reducing mortality from severe sepsis and septic shock. This involves six elements: three treatments and three tests (within the first hour).

   Tests:

- taking blood cultures to identify the type of bacteria causing sepsis
- taking a blood sample to assess the severity of sepsis
- monitoring urine output to assess kidney function

   Treatments:

- giving antibiotics
- giving fluids intravenously
- giving oxygen if levels are low (<90%)

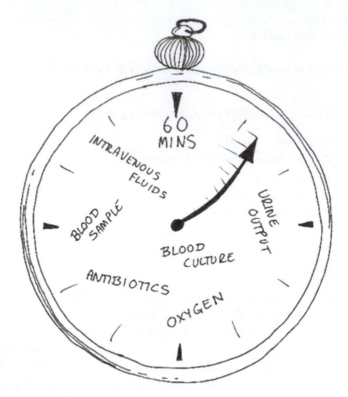

Figure 6.12   Sepsis six guidance

CHAPTER SUMMARY

- The topic of control and prevention of infection is complex.
- For those working within health and social care practice, it is essential that you not only have the skills to practise safely, but also that you understand the implications poor practice can have on the patient/service user, yourself, your employer and the wider community.
- In the ongoing fight against infection, it is essential that all working within health and social care, wherever the setting, work safely as prevention and management of infection is everyone's responsibility.

📖 FURTHER READING

Websites

Researching these websites will enhance your understanding and deepen your knowledge of the prevention and control of infection:

- Sepsis: recognition, diagnosis and early management: www.nice.org.uk/guidance/ng51
- Healthcare-associated infections: www.nice.org.uk/guidance/cg139/chapter/key-priorities-for-implementation
- About the Surviving Sepis Campaign: www.survivingsepsis.org/About-SSC/Pages/default.aspx
- Introduction to hand hygiene video: www.youtube.com/watch?v=C47vExSujVs
- NHS Improvement: www.gov.uk/government/organisations/monitor/about
- Health and Social Care Act: www.gov.uk/government/uploads/system/uploads/attachment_data/file/449049/Code_of_practice_280715_acc.pdf
- Care Quality Commission: www.cqc.org.uk/content/what-we-do
- NHS England Regional Teams: www.england.nhs.uk/about/regional-area-teams/

Books

- Tilmouth, T., Davies, E. and Williams, B. (2011) *Foundation Degree in Health and Social Care*. London: Hodder Education.
- Waugh, A. and Grant, A. (2014) *Anatomy and Physiology in Health and Illness* (12th edn). London: Churchill Livingstone.

REFERENCES

Ayliffe, G.A.J., Babb, J.R. and Quoraishi, H. (1978) A test for 'hygienic' hand disinfection. *Journal of Clinical Pathology*, 31, 923–8.

Cassini, A., Plachouras, D., Eckmanns, T., Abu Sin, M., Blank, H-P. and Ducomble, T. (2016) Burden of six healthcare-associated infections on European population health: estimating incidence-based disability-adjusted life years through a population prevalence-based modelling study. *PLOS Medicine,* 13(10): e1002150.

Department of Health (2013a) *Managing Regulated Medical Waste*. Available at: www.health.ny.gov/facilities/waste/ (accessed 10 April 2017).

Department of Health (2013b) *Health Care Waste Management Manual*. Available at: www.doh.gov.ph/sites/default/files/publications/Health_Care_Waste_Management_Manual.pdf (accessed 19 June 2017).

Department of Health (2015) *The Health and Social Care Act 2008: Code of Practice on the Prevention and Control of Infections and Related Guidance*. Available at: www.gov.uk/government/uploads/system/uploads/attachment_data/file/449049/Code_of_practice_280715_acc.pdf (accessed 17 March 2017).

Health Protection Agency (2012) *English National Point Prevalence Survey on Healthcare Associated Infections and Antimicrobial Use. 2011: Preliminary Data*. London: Health Protection Agency.

Health and Safety Executive (1992) *Personal Protective Equipment (PPE)*. Available at: www.hse.gov.uk/toolbox/ppe.htm (accessed 8 June 2017).

Health and Safety Executive (2011) *Latex Allergies in Health and Social Care*. Available at: www.hse.gov.uk/healthservices/latex/ (accessed 10 April 2017).

Loveday, H.P. (2014) Epic 3: National evidence based guidelines for preventing healthcare associated infections in NHS hospitals in England. *Journal of Hospital Infection*, 86S1, S1–S70.

NHS Choices (2017) *Benefits of Breastfeeding*. Available at: www.nhs.uk/conditions/pregnancy-and-baby/Pages/benefits-breastfeeding.aspx (accessed 13 March 2017).

Reporting of Injuries, Diseases and Dangerous Occurences Regulations 2013 (RIDDOR) Available at: www.hse.gov.uk/pubns/indg453.htm (accesed 10 April 2017).

Royal College of Nursing (2012) *Essential Practice for Infection Prevention and Control*. London: RCN.

Royal College of Nursing (2014) *The Management of Waste from Health, Social and Personal Care*. London: RCN.

The UK Sepsis Trust (2017) Available at: sepsistrust.org/ (accessed 13 March 2017).

WHO (World Health Organization) (2006) *Five Moments for Hand Hygiene*. Available at: www.who.int/gpsc/5may/background/5moments/en/ (accessed 3 October 2015).

WHO (World Health Organization) (2009) *World Health Organization Guidelines on Hand Hygiene in Healthcare. First Global Patient Safety Challenge Clean Care is Safe Care*. Geneva: WHO.

7

ESSENTIAL SKILLS FOR CARE

Gillian Rowe

I'm not telling you it's going to be easy, I'm telling you it's going to be worth it.

Art Williams

This chapter will introduce you to maths calculations in health and social care. You will also develop an understanding of the risks and hazards of clinical care and how to prepare both yourself and your patient for clinical observations. You will examine the importance of accurate record keeping and widen your knowledge of interpreting physiological measurements. This chapter is extended to include a section on medicines management, which includes medicines legislation, pharmodynamics and administration.

📌 Glossary

- **Clinical waste** This includes 'sharps', such as needles, bodily fluids and used dressings, and used PPE
- **Consent and the patient's rights** The patient's agreement to receive care, interventions and procedures
- **Contraindication** a medicine should not be used because it may be harmful to the patient
- **Drug interaction** A substance (e.g. another medicine, food) which affects the activity of a drug when both are administered together
- **Fluid balance** The measurement of fluids going into the body and fluids being excreted from the body
- **Health and Safety at Work Act 1974 (HASWA)** This legislation applies to the safety of yourself, your colleagues and the people you support
- **Indication** the use of that drug for treating a particular disease
- **Observations and physiological monitoring** Measuring vital signs
- **Pharmacodynamics** medicines which are absorbed, distributed, metabolised and excreted
- **Pharmacokinetic** medicines which act on the body

- **Pharmacology** The study of the biological effect of chemicals administered in living organisms
- **Side-effects** an effect that can be harmful or unpleasant (or occasionally beneficial)
- **Stress and resilience** The ability to deal with the pressure of working and studying

INTRODUCTION

This chapter is about the essential skills you will need in your day-to-day work: maths in calculations such as fluid balance, drug calculations, assessing risks and judging hazards with an eye on legislation and promoting good practice. All work for health and care takes place within a framework of legislation; this chapter discusses health and safety legislation applied to health and social care. This is to ensure you and your patients are kept safe when undertaking monitoring activities. You will learn how to take physiological measurements to monitor your patient's health and to aid diagnosis. These skills need to be practised under supervision until you have been assessed competent to practise. Developing clinical skills is hard work, but as retired American billionaire Art Williams (above) states, it is worth the effort. The more confident you are in your skills, the more effective you will be in your practice.

WHY DO WE USE MATHS IN HEALTH AND SOCIAL CARE?

It is probable that you have already undertaken functional skills level 3 or GCSE maths. Many students will have struggled with abstract ideas such as algebra (something you will use if you specialise in orthopaedic trauma), fractions and percentages. However, you will be using maths regularly in your day-to-day work. Here are a few examples to remind you and some drug calculations to work through.

[1] Mrs Jones is on a strict fluid balance chart. Today she had IV fluids 1300 ml and oral fluids 450 ml. Her catheter bag contained 1250 ml, she vomited twice today, judged approximately 200ml, her wound drainage bag contained 50 ml. What was her fluid balance total?

IN	OUT
1300 ml	200 ml
450 ml	1250 ml
	50 ml
1750 ml	1500 ml

[2] Mr Smith weighed 76.20 kg when he was admitted to your unit, he now weighs 74.18 kg. How much weight has he lost?

76.20
−74.18
‾‾‾‾‾‾
2.02 kg

You might have to convert stones and pounds into kilos. Table 7.1 gives you the formula for this.

Table 7.1   Converting stones to kilograms

1 stone (14 pounds)	6.35 kilograms
1 pound	0.45 of a kilogram
1 kilogram	2.2 pounds (approximately)

Drug calculations

[1] Mrs Baker is taking OxyNorm liquid (OxyContin) 5 milligrams (mg) (dose) in 5 millilitres (ml) (volume) of liquid for pain relief. She can take 2.5 mg every 3 hours. What is her maximum total dose in any 24 hours?

$24 \div 3 = 8$

$8 \times 2.5 = 20$ mg/ml daily total

[2] Mrs Jones weighs 14 stone (88.90 kg). Her medication dose is 2.5 micrograms (mcg) per kilo, how many micrograms should she receive?

88.90 kg

$\times 2.5$

222.25 mcg

You need to ensure that you know the conversions for micrograms, milligrams and grams. Table 7.2 gives you these.

Table 7.2   Converting micrograms to grams

1,000,000 micrograms (mcg)	1 gram(g)
1,000 micrograms (mcg)	1 milligram (mg)
1,000 milligrams (mg)	1 gram (g)

[3] Mr Turner needs 6 milligrams of his medication, but the stock cupboard has only 10 milligrams (dose) in 5 millilitres (volume). What volume are you going to give him?

$$\frac{\text{Dose required}}{\text{Dose available}} \times \frac{\text{Volume}}{1} = \frac{6}{10} \times \frac{5}{1} = 3 \text{ millilitres}$$

The NHS uses a mnemonic called 'Need and Have' to help you will this:

$$\frac{\text{Need}}{\text{Have}} \times \frac{\text{Strength}}{1}$$

So, Mrs Jones needs 250 mg of penicillin and the stock cupboard has 125 mg tablets in 125 mg strength:

$$\frac{\text{Need } 250 \text{ mg}}{\text{Have } 125 \text{ mg}} \times \frac{\text{Strength } 125 \text{ mg}}{1} = 2 \text{ tablets}$$

If you struggle with fractions, download an app to your phone and practise doing them. If you are not sure, *always* get someone to check your calculation, it is better to be safe than sorry. Look at Table 7.3 and ensure that these never events do not happen.

Table 7.3   Safety first: never events

Always check you have the right patient, the right medication and the right dose
Never give someone another patient's drugs, even if they are the same dose
Never cut tablets into 2, even if they are scored and you have a pill cutter

HEALTH AND SAFETY AT WORK

What is a risk and what is a hazard?

A hazard is an object that can potentially do harm, and risk is the likelihood of harm occurring. Health and social care work is classed as a hazardous occupation due to the nature of the work. The potential for infection is high. The latest figures available from the Health and Safety Executive (HSE) state 'infection rates of about 30 per 100,000 workers per year amongst nurses and about 100 per 100,000 per year amongst care workers in residential homes' (HSE, 2016). There were about 5 million lost working days (1.78 days per worker) due to work-related illness and injury in the health and social care sector. This is one of the highest levels in any employment sector. Chapter 6, Prevention and Control of Infection, gives greater detail on self-protection.

Employers and employees must abide by the Health and Safety at Work Act 1974 (HASWA) and its many amendments and regulations by providing you with a safe working environment, protective equipment and health and safety training. Employers or their designated persons must carry out risk assessments, and put control measures in place to reduce risks to all people who use, visit or work in their setting. You, as an employee, are obligated to take reasonable care of yourself and others, and not put yourself or others at risk by your actions or inactions, and you must cooperate with your employer on health and safety matters.

Your employer should risk assess procedures and produce guidance for you to follow. You should understand these protocols are there to protect you and your patients. However, you too should risk assess each activity to ensure you are engaging in safe working practice and are monitoring the risk and modifying the process if it is needed.

Legislation

Control of risk from biohazardous agents rests with the employer but each employee is bound by the Control of Substances Hazardous to Health 2002 (COSSH) legislation. Patients are at risk from care workers through healthcare-associated infections (HAIs) (see Chapter 6), especially now that so many infectious agents are becoming resistant to antibiotics.

Staff are at great risk of needlestick injuries and attention needs to be paid when drawing up, giving and removing needles. It is easy to be distracted and then accidents happen. Safe disposal of used needles and syringes should be in accordance with infection control protocols; they are usually put into a sharps box. The most common risks of sharps contamination are hepatitis B (HBV), hepatitis C (HCV) and human immunodeficiency virus (HIV). HSE (2016) states that 'four health workers have died after having accidentally incurred needlestick injuries during work with HIV patients. Another nine are also known to be sero-positive because of this kind of accident.'

Any workplace accidents need to be recorded and reported under the Reporting of Injuries, Diseases and Dangerous Occurrences Regulations 2013 (RIDDOR). The forms used are provided by HSE and this is a legal document which is submissible in a court of law.

Staff are also at risk when moving and handling patients. You should receive special training to prevent damage both to yourself and your patients (Manual Handling Operations Regulations 1992). Legislation in the form of the Provision and Use of Work Equipment Regulations 1998 (PUWER) and the Lifting Operations and Lifting Equipment Regulations 1998 (LOLER) are regulations to support safe working practice. You should never undertake the use of mechanical lifting equipment until you have received training on each piece of equipment and, if relevant, how to use and check slings. You will also need training for safe manual handling and the use of such aids as transfer belts and sliding sheets. Read Scenario 7.1 and think about how correct attention to health and safety could have prevented this incident.

 Scenario 7.1

Mr Robinson has an acquired brain injury after being in a traumatic road traffic event (RTE). He is very restless and at risk of falling out of bed. A risk assessment was undertaken and cot sides were installed on his bed.

The assessment considered:

- the rail is suitable for the bed and mattress
- the mattress fits snugly between the rails
- the rail is correctly fitted, secure and will be regularly inspected and maintained
- gaps that could cause entrapment of neck, head and chest have been eliminated

Staff on the unit were trained in the use of bedrails and a daily check list was instituted.

(Continued)

(Continued)

Mr Robinson was later assessed as at risk of developing pressure ulcers and it was decided to put an air wave overlay mattress on the bed. This should have triggered a new risk assessment for his cot sides as Mr Robinson is now higher in the bed.

During the night, Mr Robinson rolled over the cot sides and sustained a fractured neck of femur and bruising to his torso.

Bedrails are classed as medical devices, which fall under the authority of the Medicines and Healthcare Products Regulatory Agency (MHRA) and HSE was informed of this event.

Go Further 7.1

Type 'bedrail assessment' into a search engine and you will find free resources which are useful in ensuring that you understand safe practice with bedrails. If your patients use bedrails in your care facility, ask for training to assess the bedrails and ensure that you have a recording method in place for monitoring their safety.

Dealing with violence at work

Sadly, violence is increasing in health and social care settings, and is never acceptable. Your employer should give you training on how to prevent workplace harassment or violence. Quite often, people who are anxious or in pain become aggressive and by using clear communication, the threat of violence can be removed.

Go Further 7.2

Read the advice given in the Royal College of Nursing 'Violence at work' booklet on the RCN website.

Dealing with stress

Work-related stress develops because a person is unable to cope with the demands being placed on them. The latest statistics show that the total number of cases of work-related stress, depression or anxiety in 2014/15 was 440,000 cases, a prevalence rate of 1,380 per 100,000 workers who have reported suffering from stress (HSE, 2016).

Some kinds of stress are useful (eustress); this is the kind of stress that gets things done (such as last-minute essay writing), however, too much stress leads to distress, which if it is prolonged, can lead to depression and anxiety. Coming to work when ill (so called presenteeism) can create an even bigger burden than sickness absence from work. However, fear of losing your job or the fear that absence will negatively affect your career prospects adds to the stress burden. This is a harsh judgement call at a time when you don't need it.

Developing resilience

Learning how to manage your workload and prioritise is an essential skill when studying and working in the health and social care sector. Care work itself is stressful: when helping people who are suffering, we sometimes over identify with our patients and take their suffering personally. You have to learn to switch off and if that is difficult, use your reflective journal (you can find more about journal keeping in Chapter 3, Personal and Professional Development) as a place to record your feelings regarding the day's events. This will give you the opportunity to consider why you feel the way you do at a later, calmer moment. You can read more about resilience in Chapter 4, Leadership and Teamwork in Health and Social Care.

PATIENTS' RIGHTS

Before you undertake any activity with your patient, you must receive consent. Patients have fundamental legal and ethical rights to determine what happens to their own bodies; also, seeking consent is a matter of common curtesy. Discuss what you are going to do and say why you need to do it. Explain carefully, using language the patient understands. Remember that consent must be voluntary and informed. If the activity is going to be uncomfortable, say so, don't lie, or imply the patient is being difficult if they complain they are uncomfortable. If patients are properly prepared, they are more likely to give consent.

When taking repeated observations or measurements, ask for consent each time, do not assume that agreeing to the procedure once is an implicit consent for continued observations or measurements.

If the patient is incapable of giving consent, remember that any activities should be in their 'best interests', and you should seek permission (preferably written and recorded) from a family member or mental capacity advocate. Table 7.4 tells you who can give consent.

Table 7.4   What is consent and who can give it

The parents of a child under the age of 14
A child of 14 or over who is assessed as 'Gillick competent'
Any adult over the age of 18 has a right under common law to grant or withhold consent to examination/investigation or treatment, except in certain special circumstances, such as those with a community treatment order (CTO) under the Mental Health Act 2008
Competent adults also have a right to refuse procedures or treatment for reasons that are 'rational, irrational or for no reason'
Consent must not be induced by force or fraud, neither must the withholding or withdrawing of consent during an examination, investigation or treatment affect the quality of care the patient receives.

Covert drug administration

Both the Nursing and Midwifery Council (NMC) and the Royal College of Physicians (RCP) have a position on covert administration and are guided by the Mental Capacity Act 2005. The patient has the right to refuse medication. However, distinctions need to be made between those who would not know they were taking medication 'and others who would be aware if they were not deceived into thinking otherwise' (NMC, 2016). Accordingly, the RCP (2016) states 'Treatment should be made available to severely incapacitated individuals judged in their best interests and administered in the least restrictive manner, and in exceptional circumstances it may be necessary to administer medication in foodstuffs without the individual's awareness that it is being done'. Therefore, when considering disguising medication, the treatment must be necessary to save life, prevent deterioration and ensure improvement in the individual's physical and mental health.

MAKING CLINICAL OBSERVATIONS AND MONITORING VITAL SIGNS

Health and nutrition

It is important to monitor your patients' weight (see below) but you should also monitor what they are eating and record their daily consumption. For this you could use a Malnutrition Universal Screening Tool (MUST). Quite often, obese or underweight adults are suffering from malnutrition either because they are not eating enough or because they are eating cheap energy-dense foods that lack vital nutrients. Poor-quality foods can affect the patient's immune system which can impair wound healing and delay recovery (see Chapter 5, Bioscience, for more detail). Excess weight can promote type 2 diabetes and add to the risk of developing heart disease, being overweight can also lead to depression and poor self-image which can lead to self-neglect. Activity 7.1 shows you how to calculate someone's BMI using different methods.

Nutritional support may be needed if the patient has issues with swallowing. This can include thickening agents, soft diet, or artificial feeding systems such as enteral or parenteral nutrition.

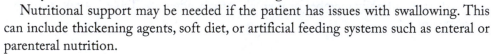 Activity 7.1

To calculate a BMI:

- First: divide your weight in kilograms (kg) by your height in metres (m)
- Then: divide the answer by your height again to get your BMI.

$$BMI = \frac{Weight\ (kg)}{Height\ (m)^2}$$

A BMI in the 20–25 range is desirable, below 18 is underweight and over 30 is very obese. For example, Mrs Brown is 5 foot 2 inches tall and weighs 12 stone. What is her BMI?

Change her weight and height into metric:

> Height: 5 ft 2inches = 1.72 metres
>
> Weight: 12 stone = 168lbs = 76.2 kg
>
> Therefore: 76.2 ÷1.72 = 44.3
>
> 44.3 ÷1.72 = 25.7 therefore her BMI is 25.7

If the patient does not know their height or weight, or is unable to communicate, you can estimate their BMI by taking a measurement of their mid-arm circumference. If it is greater than 32 cm they are likely to be overweight, if it is under 23 cm, they are likely to be underweight.

Limitations of BMI

Measuring BMI is a good indicator but it does have its limitations, especially with athletes and for the elderly. For athletes, a BMI may overestimate the amount of fat and for the elderly it may underestimate the amount of fat due to muscle loss. Measuring waist circumference helps screen for possible health risks that come with obesity, therefore measuring waist and hips can give a better indication of health risk: a waist size that is greater than 35 inches for women or greater than 40 inches for men can indicate a risk of type 2 diabetes and heart disease.

Preparing for observation

When you first see your patient, employ what has been called 'the medical gaze' (Foucault, 1963). This is looking for 'telling signs' and reading your patient's body language. Look at their demeanour (sad, tired, happy, in pain, tearful), the way they sit or lie, their skin colour (pallor, flushed, sweaty).

Recent weight loss or gain can be judged by looking at the patient's clothing: is it loose or tight? Look at the patient's hands, are rings loose or tight?

They may have been neglecting themselves, do they look clean and well cared for or do their clothes look unkempt? Do they smell unpleasantly, is their hair clean and brushed?

What about their breath? Have they cleaned their teeth or dentures? Breath smelling of acetone (smells like they have been sucking pear drops) can indicate diabetes.

Are their eyes red rimmed and rheumy, are the whites red? They may have an eye infection.

When you speak to the patient, ask how they are, does their response match your summation of their condition? Quite often people will try to put on a brave face, they don't like to be a bother or feel embarrassed if they need pain relief, or need help with an activity they can normally do themselves.

Preparing the environment

Ensure the area is private to maintain the patient's dignity, quiet, free from draughts, is well lit and that the patient is comfortable. Also, check the area is free from risks or hazards to you and the patient. You have responsibilities under the Health and Safety at Work Act 1974. Table 7.5 tells you what some of these are.

Table 7.5   Health and Safety at Work Act 1974 (HASWA)

Take reasonable care for your own health and safety and to others who may be affected by what you do or do not do
Cooperate with your employer on health and safety
Correctly use work items provided by your employer, including personal protective equipment, in accordance with training or instructions
Do not interfere with or misuse anything provided for your health and safety or welfare

Source: hse.gov.uk, 2016

Preparing yourself

Physical contact with patients carries risk of contamination and therefore you need to be wearing **personal protective equipment** (PPE) (see also Chapter 6). Your employer must provide such things as single use vinyl gloves and aprons. Some organisations still use latex gloves but these are being phased out due to the number of allergies they provoke in staff. In order to reduce cross-infection and contamination, it is vital that you use PPE and change it every time you move on to another patient. You may need to wear a face mask and gown if the patient is infectious and in some cases white boots need to be worn too. Depending on the patient's condition, these may be kept inside their room if you are 'barrier nursing' (protecting yourself from the patient) or outside their room if you are 'reverse barrier' nursing (protecting the patient from you).

Ensure that you have a nurse's fob watch (cheap from Amazon/eBay and some organisations give them away free). Some watches can be removed from the rubber or plastic case so that the case can be cleaned to reduce the risk of cross-infection. Please do not use your mobile phone as a timing device as it will become a source of contamination and you will put yourself and anyone else who uses your phone at risk.

Hand washing is critical to infection control. Chapter 6, Prevention and Control of Infection, goes into this in greater detail and describes the correct six-step procedure (see Figure 6.4). It also discusses use of cleansing gels, but remember they are not a substitute for hand washing, but complementary to washing. Wash your hands before and after any patient contact (Table 7.6).

Your employer also should provide 'clinical hazard' bags (usually bright yellow) for you to place used PPE in. These bags need to be collected by a specialist company who

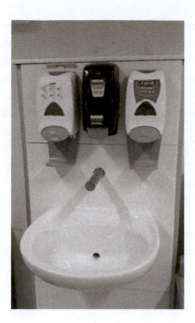

Figure 7.1   Washing your hands

Table 7.6	Hand washing: Remember …
Before doing anything.....Wash your hands After doing anything.........Wash your hands And wear PPE	

are licensed by the local authority to dispose of the contents safely. The bags therefore need to be stored safely until collection.

Preparing the equipment

Make sure you have enough space and the right resources to undertake the measurement and that any electrical equipment you are using has been recently PAT tested (PAT = Portable Appliance Testing) and is functioning. If it is battery powered, ensure you have spare batteries in case of malfunction, or that it has been properly charged and has been stored in a safe place. Any broken or faulty equipment must be reported as soon as possible, and a faulty sign appended to it to warn others.

Preparing the patient

Prior to your measuring their vital signs, the patient should have the opportunity to sit for approximately 5 minutes to calm them down, especially if you have asked the patient to walk from one area to another. This will allow their blood pressure to resolve while they are resting and give an accurate resting pulse. If you leave the patient to rest, ensure that you come back within 10 minutes at the most. Any longer than that and the patient may become anxious as they will think they have been forgotten, which could give misleading high blood pressure results.

The patient should be asked to, or assisted to, loosen clothing or remove arm coverings (cardigans/jumpers) ready for you to take their blood pressure. Also, if you are taking the patient's blood pressure, ensure they visit the toilet first, as a full bladder increases blood pressure and can give a false reading. The patient should be sitting comfortably and not on the edge of a bed if there is a risk of falling. Ensure that you remember the 4 Rs before you begin taking the observations:

- **Respect** the patient's dignity and privacy
- **Reassure** the patient in a manner that minimises fears or concerns
- **Record** the results
- **Report** any concerns

Measuring vital signs

Physiological measurements are an important part of your caring role because they allow the patient's condition to be monitored and ensure prompt detection of adverse events or developing conditions.

What is normal?

Biomarker measurement ranges are arrived at by taking mass measurements and arriving at a median. For instance: normal temperature (98.4°F/36°C) was determined by Carl Wunderlich (in the early nineteenth century) by taking the temperature of 25,000 patients. He also noted that normal temperature varies through the circadian cycle, and is consistently lower in older individuals – something that is not always acknowledged when considering fever in the elderly.

Pain

Pain is not a normal daily event and is always an indicator that something is not right, therefore any pain is abnormal and is an indicator of the presence of an ailment. Patients should be assessed for the presence of pain and it should be treated promptly and effectively. It can adversely affect measurement accuracy in the same way that anxiety can, possibly leading to a misdiagnosis.

Weight

Patients should be weighed when they enter your setting, and they should be weighed each month to monitor their overall health. Weight loss or gain can be indicative of an underlying health issue which can be psychological and physical. Unplanned weight loss is an acute risk factor and may indicate an underlying health condition.

Measurement of physiological parameters

The NEWS (National Early Warning Score) chart (Table 7.7) has replaced previous recording charts as it is more dynamic in assisting diagnosis. It is traffic light colour coded showing warning (amber) and danger (red) areas which should alert you to a patient's condition. This gives an aggregated score showing areas of risk. A downloadable version of the NEWS chart can be found at www.rcplondon.ac.uk/projects/outputs/national-early-warning-score-news.

Table 7.7   National Early Warning Scores (NEWS)

The physiological parameters which form the basis of the scoring system are:

1   Respiratory rate
2   Oxygen saturations
3   Temperature
4   Systolic blood pressure
5   Pulse rate
6   Level of consciousness

Temperature

The normal body temperature of a person varies depending on gender, recent activity, food and fluid consumption, time of day, and for women, the stage of the menstrual cycle. Older people or people with disabilities that restrict movement have a lower 'normal or usual' temperature. It is important that you understand what temperature is. It also changes depending on the site in the body where the reading is taken. A rectal reading will be higher than one take in the axilla (armpit). Therefore, when taking a reading it is important to be consistent in the chosen site (oral, aural, rectal, axillary). Aural thermometers quite often have single use plastic covers to prevent cross infection and these are to be preferred where possible. Tempa-dot thermometers are single use and need to be disposed of safely and to company convention.

It is also important to use the same device to ensure accuracy, whether it is a digital or chemical tool, as the reading will differ by as much as a degree. Some settings use liquid crystal scan strips which are placed on the forehead; while these are safer than glass thermometers, they are not known for their accuracy, whereas the Tempa-dot chemical thermometers are more accurate than the strips, but not as accurate as an aural or rectal thermometer.

The body temperature is generated by heat produced through movement and metabolic activity, it is regulated in the hypothalamus area of the brain and informed by thermoreceptors in muscles, the liver and sensory receptors in the peripheral nervous system. Thermoregulation is a negative feedback system and is one of the functions of homeostasis.

When preparing to take the temperature, do not do it after the patient has just had a hot or chilled drink, smoked a cigarette, had a hot bath/shower or engaged in moderate/vigorous exercise as this will give a false high or low reading, which can lead to an incorrect diagnosis and inappropriate treatment. An inaccurate reading will also be given if you do not leave the thermometer in place for long enough, or in the case of a tympanic thermometer, not insert it correctly. Look at Table 7.8 to see what is normal and abnormal temperature.

Table 7.8   Temperature gradients

Normal temperature	36-37.5°C
Hyperthermia	< 35°C
Low grade pyrexia	37.5-38°C
Moderate to high pyrexia	38-40°C
Hyperpyrexia	40+°C

Pulse

The pulse is the pressure wave of blood moving through pliable arteries, and a reading can be taken at pulse points where an artery passes over a bone. This is a fairly accurate way to assess the condition of the heart and circulatory system. The reading will indicate the number of heart beats, and can also be used to examine the strength of the beat (full and bounding/weak and thready) and the regularity of the beat. Various machines can count the pulse but they cannot give this additional information, so it is always useful to do a manual pulse check as well as a digital reading.

Compress the chosen artery with two fingers, ease off the pressure slightly as you do not want to cut off the blood flow, and using a watch, time your count for a full 60 seconds. This will give you the resting heart rate. Table 7.9 gives the range of pulse rates.

The pulse rate changes often and rapidly. It is affected by caffeine, smoking, exercise, stress, anxiety, fever, weight and medication.

Table 7.9   Pulse rates

	Beats per minutes
Babies	100-160
Young children	60-140
Adolescents and adults	60-80
Athletes	40-60
Bradycardia	Less than 60
Tachycardia	More than 100

Respiration

Breathing is the act of inhaling oxygen-rich air and exhaling carbon-dioxide-rich air. Oxygen is attached to red blood cells in the alveoli of the lungs for transportation around the body and is then used in cellular respiration. Pulse and respiration are related because the heart and lungs work together. Normally, an increase or decrease in one causes the same effect on the other.

Observing someone breathing can lead to them breathing more rapidly, so try to be surreptitious about it. There isn't a machine that can do this, so you must practise breathing observation and counting breaths over a minute by watching the patient's chest rise and fall. Note that *one breath = breathing in and out.*

Respiration rates may increase with fever, also note whether a person has any difficulty breathing such as dyspnoea, stridor, stertor (while sleeping), wheezing, rasping, or chest noises that could indicate a chest infection, asthma, bronchitis or COPD (chronic obstructive pulmonary disease – emphysema). Table 7.10 gives the range of respiration rates.

Table 7.10   Respiration rates

Normal breathing rate at rest	16–20 breaths per minute
Abnormal breathing rate at rest	Under 12 breaths or over 25

Oxygen saturation

Pulse oximetry is a non-invasive method of monitoring the percentage of haemoglobin that is saturated with oxygen. The device clips onto a finger (toe or earlobe) (see Figure 7.2) using red and infrared light, and measures the amount of oxygen in the blood. Red blood cells must carry sufficient oxygen through the arteries to all of the internal organs to keep you alive. Normally, when red blood cells pass through the lungs, 95-100% of them are saturated with oxygen. If someone has lung disease or anaemia, fewer of the red blood cells may be carrying their usual load of oxygen, and

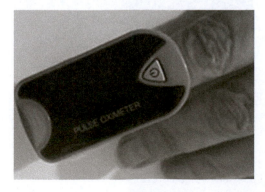

Figure 7.2   Pulse oximeter

the oxygen saturation level might be lower than 95%. If the reading is below 90%, the patient will need oxygen support. These machines often will give a pulse reading also. It is important to note that the machines use red and infrared light waves and they cannot work if the patient has nail varnish on their fingers or toes.

Blood pressure

This measures the force of the blood pushing against the artery walls. Each time the heart beats, it pumps blood into the arteries. Blood pressure is therefore usually measured in the left arm as the brachial artery is nearest to the heart, although the right arm and the legs can be used if necessary. Blood pressure is measured in millimetres of mercury (mmHg). Blood pressure is affected by caffeine, smoking, exercise, stress, fever, weight, salt intake, alcohol, age, heart disease and medication.

- The force of contraction in the ventricles is called the **systolic** rate
- The resting heart pressure is called the **diastolic** rate

⚙️ Activity 7.2

Practise taking a blood pressure reading. Raise the person's arm so that the brachial artery is roughly at the same height as the heart. If the arm is held too high, the reading will be artificially lowered, and vice versa. Ensure that the arm and back are supported and the feet are resting firmly on the floor, not dangling.

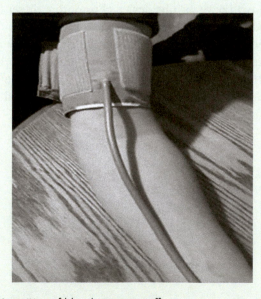

Figure 7.3   Correct position of blood pressure cuff

The cuff should be applied directly over the skin (tight or thick clothes artificially raise blood pressure). Position the lower cuff border 2.5 cm above the bend in the elbow so the inflatable bladder is over the brachial artery (Figure 7.3). Correct positioning is important to the accuracy of the reading and for the comfort of the patient. Ensure that you use the correct cuff size for the patient.

Usually, blood pressure is measured using digital machines but it is always useful to know how to take a manual BP. The cuff is placed on the arm as described above, ensuring the bend in the arm is exposed. Inflate the bladder on the cuff to 10% over the last reading, or 160 mmHG. A stethoscope is placed over the antecubital fossa to listen for the blood flow, known as the Korotkoff sounds:

I   Systolic pressure – tapping sound – take reading

II   Sounds become fainter

Auscultatory gap – sounds may disappear

III   Return of clear sounds – diastolic pressure – take a reading

IV   Muffling

V   Sounds completely disappear

Table 7.11 gives the range of blood pressure readings

Table 7.11   Blood pressure

Normal systolic pressure: which is the heart contracting	120–139 mmHg
Normal diastolic pressure: which is the heart resting	60–89 mmHg
Hypertension	140/90 mmHg or higher
Hypotension	90/60 mmHg or lower

Postural hypotension

If the patient suffers from dizziness or fainting when arising, they may have postural hypotension. Postural measurements may be used to determine if postural dizziness (feeling dizzy when standing up) is the result of a fall in blood pressure.

First measure the BP when the patient is supine (lying down) and then repeat it after the patient has stood for 2 minutes, which allows for equilibration. The patient may need to be supported, with their arm held in the correct position, and if using a digital cuff, someone should hold this in the correct position too.

Neurological assessment: levels of consciousness

Assessing the level consciousness of your patient is part of critical clinical care, and considers the degree of arousal and awareness. Causes of loss of consciousness include: lack of oxygen (hypoxia), stroke, analgesia, overdose (drugs and alcohol), sedatives and subarachnoid haemorrhage. The pupil size and reactivity can indicate arousal or brain injury. When assessing a patient's response to verbal stimulus, it is helpful to know if they have a hearing loss. The states of consciousness are given in Table 7.12.

Table 7.12   Levels of consciousness

1. Alert and awake
2. Confusion: Not orientated to time and space
3. Lethargy: Sleepy but can be roused
4. Obtundation: Extreme drowsiness, difficult to rouse
5. Stupor: No response other than to painful stimuli
6. Comatose: No response

The quick system of AVPU can be used to judge the appropriate response:

A = alert

V = responds to vocal prompts

P = responds to painful stimulus

U = unresponsive

If the patient is unresponsive then an assessment tool such as the Glasgow Coma Scale can be used to gauge the depth of unconsciousness.

Pressure area risk assessment

Patients need to be assessed for pressure areas. There are several tools available for this, such as the Waterlow Score or the Braden Score, and your employer will have a record of which score tool is used. The purpose of the scoring system is to inform you if your patient is at risk of developing pressure sores (decubitus ulcers) and to develop a plan of care which prevents this from happening. In nearly all instances of pressure area ulcers, poor nursing care is the cause. Patients of ethnic origin with darker skin are just as much at risk of developing pressure ulcers but sometimes the signs are missed.

Remember when assessing darkly pigmented skin that it does not blanch, but may be violaceous (eggplant colour) or purplish blue.

Pressure ulcers occur when the patient cannot move or reposition themselves in the bed (or chair), usually because they are acutely ill, malnourished or have mobility issues such as stroke or paralysis. Some elderly people or patients who are obese may have difficulty in moving around in bed and therefore are at risk. Pressure ulcers are painful and they can take a long time to heal and this negatively affects the quality of life of the patient.

The patient's skin should be assessed, especially if they are incontinent, underweight (have bony prominences) and lack mobility. The heels, shoulders and sacrum need regular observation and any redness in the skin needs early preventative treatment. Pressure ulcers can also occur on the back of the head and the ears.

Young children who are receiving intervention such as nasogastric feeding or in splints or casts also need regular observation to prevent such ulcers occurring.

In the event of a pressure ulcer forming, a specialist tissue viability nurse should be consulted and advice taken as to the type of wound and wound dressing to be used. Care providers should know that pressure sores above grade 3 need to be reported to the CQC (Care Quality Commission).

Preparing the patient at the end of observation

Assist the patient to redress and to return to their chair or bed, if you have moved them. Explain the results: it is not enough to give a generic or soothing answer, if someone has an elevated temperature (hyperthermia/pyrexia), say so and offer a homely remedy such as a cooling drink, and thank them for their cooperation.

Ensure that you clean any equipment used by wiping it down with products recommended by your employer's convention and replace equipment in a safe place. If need be, put it back on charge in order that it is ready to be used again. Dispose of your PPE to convention and wash your hands thoroughly.

Urinalysis

Normal urine is pale straw colour (may be darker in the morning), has a non-offensive odour and should be clear with nothing floating in it.

[1] Ensure safe working practice and wear personal protective clothing, disposable gloves and apron.
[2] Collect urine in a clean, dry, covered container and test it as soon as possible.
[3] If testing cannot be done within 2 hours after voiding, refrigerate the specimen immediately for preservation. Do not use a domestic refrigerator used for food.
[4] Allow the urine specimen to return to room temperature prior to testing.

To carry out the test you will need: a box of in-date reagent strips, a timing device and a paper towel (Figure 7.4).

Labelling samples

Always label the sample pot in the room you took the sample or at the bedside as this reduces the risk of errors.

Always confirm the patient's name and date of birth before removing the specimen from the room (even if it is someone you know very well).

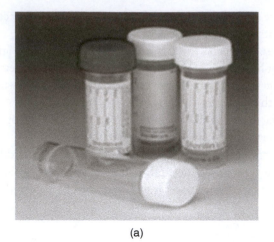
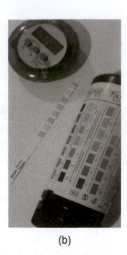

(a)   (b)

Figure 7.4   (a) Urine sample containers (b) Preparing to test urine

Testing urine

[1] Remove one reagent strip from the bottle and replace the cap immediately.
[2] Completely immerse reagent areas of the strip in FRESH urine and remove immediately to avoid dissolving out reagents.
[3] Ensure all of the test pads are wet.
[4] After dipping, run the edge of the entire length of the strip against the rim of the urine container to remove excess urine.
[5] Hold the strip in a horizontal position to prevent possible mixing of chemicals from adjacent reagent areas and/or contaminating the hands with urine.
[6] Blot the strip to remove excess urine by touching the edge to a paper towel. Do not drag the strip across the towel; touch the edge only.

Remember to hold the strip vertically and the bottle horizontally to compare colour readings (Figure 7.5). Ensure no urine comes into contact with the bottle.

Proper read time is critical for an optimal result. The side of the bottle will tell you the time for each reading.

Dispose of the stick per health and safety rules/company convention. Table 7.13 gives you the signs and symptoms of a urinary tract infection (UTI).

Stool examination

The Bristol Stool Chart (Figure 7.6) is pictorial and gives an explanation of what different types of faeces can indicate. Stools are typed 1–7 from hard and compacted to liquid. The stool chart offers diagnostic assistance by suggesting causes and outcomes if the situation is not remedied. For instance, hard and compacted faeces can be caused by poor diet, low fluid intake and a lack of exercise, the passage of such faeces can damage the lining of the bowel and cause ano-rectal bleeding due to laceration. The exertion of trying to excrete such faeces might cause the development of haemorrhoids (piles), which are swollen blood vessels in the anus.

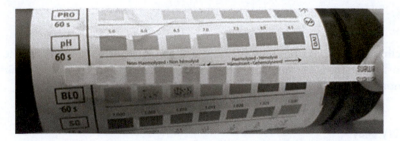

Figure 7.5   Can you spot the mistake?

Table 7.13   Signs and symptoms of a urinary tract infection

Pain on passing urine – burning/stinging sensation
Low abdominal pain
Urine frequency
Urine appearing abnormal – colour, clarity, odour
High temperature
Confusion

	BRISTOL STOOL CHART		
	Type 1	Separate hard lumps	Very constipated
	Type 2	Lumpy and sausage like	Slightly constipated
	Type 3	A sausage shape with cracks in the surface	Normal
	Type 4	Like a smooth, soft sausage or snake	Normal
	Type 5	Soft blobs with clear-cut edges	Lacking fibre
	Type 6	Mushy consistency with ragged edges	Inflammation
	Type 7	Liquid consistency with no solid pieces	Inflammation

Figure 7.6   The Bristol stool chart

RECORDING AND REPORTING

Ensure that you chart the results and report any concerns to your senior staff member. Recording results is critical to understanding your patient's health. Gaps in charts lead to frustration by the medical team as they may be making a diagnosis and offering interventions based on misleading or incorrect information.

Residential care settings need to take baseline measurements at least monthly in order to have a good understanding of the general health of their patients, and this should include recording their patients' weight too, to ensure that weight gain or loss is being monitored.

ESSENTIAL SKILLS: MEDICINES MANAGEMENT AND ADMINISTRATION

The clinical, cost-effective and safe use of medicines to ensure patients get the maximum benefit from the medicines they need, whilst at the same time minimising potential harm. (MHRA, 2014)

Regulatory body

Medicines management law is The Human Medicines Regulations (2012), which gives the scope, provisions and classifications of medicinal products and gives the regulations for prescribing and pharmaceutical practice (among many other things). The Medicines & Healthcare products Regulatory Agency (MHRA) regulates medicines, medical devices and blood components for transfusion and oversees the issuing of yellow cards and adverse warnings, it also hosts various advisory committees and The Clinical Practice Datalink (CPRD) database and the National Institute for Biological Standards and Control (NIBSC), Go Further 7.18 gives the links for further investigation.

Go Further 7.18

www.gov.uk/government/organisations/medicines-and-healthcare-products-regulatory-agency/about

Medicines optimisation guide from NICE https://www.nice.org.uk/guidance/ng5

How do medicines work?

Medication can be delivered orally (and sub-lingual), aurally, rectally (PR), in the vagina (PV), optically, nasally, rubbed in, injected, implanted, and trans dermally. It can also be administered through cannula and drips. The chosen route affects absorption, distribution, metabolism and elimination (ADME). Routes are chosen depending on the tissue being targeted, severity of illness, urgency of the problem and the patient's general state of health.

Medication is **absorbed** via the bloodstream to the liver where drug metabolism occurs (the first-pass effect), the drug metabolites may be more or less potent and may pass through the liver several times before being eliminated. Capsulated oral medication is protected from gastric acid and releases the dose into the intestine for absorption. Dissolved drug metabolites are **distributed** into the cells and function through biochemical reactions, they then pass back to the liver, are **metabolically** deactivated and then **excreted**.

The brain is generally protected from drug activity by the brain-blood barrier unless the brain has inflammation, in which case, large molecule antibiotics can pass through (see Chapter 5, Bioscience and Chapter 6, The Control and Prevention of Infection). Some medication is designed to take advantage of weakness in the blood-brain barrier (such as L Dopa), these need to be fat soluble to be effective. Neurotransmitters can be modified by specific psychoactive substances such as opiates and Benzodiazepines acting on cell receptors.

Pharmacodynamics

Most drugs either inhibit or mimic physiological/biochemical actions or patho-logical processes by depressing or stimulating agonist receptors. The binding of drugs (ligands) requires numerous biomolecular processes. Absorption rates vary with age, weight, fat and muscle mass and delivery system, also the time the drug is taken such as before/after/with food will also have an impact on metabolism and elimination, thus pharmacokinetics seeks to understand the interactions between drugs and the biological environment (such as between the bloodstream and oily cell surfaces) in order to predict the bioavailability (the therapeutic window) of the drug. This was first understood by Claude Bernard in the 1880's when he discovered how Curare causes paralysis by blocking the neurotransmitter acetylcholine. Some drugs can be considered broad spectrum as they can fit into many cell receptors (and thus possibly cause side effects). Occasionally, metabolism causes an inactive compound to become pharmacologically active, or innocuous drugs to create a toxic chemical.

There is a correlation between the quantity of drug administered and the drug response (the dose-effect relationship), all drugs have a threshold range where the intended effect is greater than unintended effect (side effects). Those with narrow ther-apeutic ranges are difficult to manage and need frequent monitoring (such as thyroxine and digoxin) pharmacologists use blood (and urine) to calculate drug processing time and adjust dosage accordingly.

Medication is graded into 3 main categories according to The Medicines Act 1968:

1. General sales list (GSL)
2. Pharmacy only (Pharmacist must be present)
3. Prescription only (POM) (Pharmacist only to dispense)

Drugs used in the UK are collated into The British National Formulary (BNF) and is a pharmaceutical reference book, it is published twice per year (March and September) and gives information by detailing all medicines that are prescribed in the UK; the box below explains the information given. It is used by all healthcare professionals as a reference for prescribing and information.

> Indications – what the drug is used for
> Dosages – mg, drops, tabs, puffs
> Contraindications – when not to give
> Cautions – give with care
> Side effects – unwanted effects
> Interaction – with other drugs or food

Legislation

Medication is prescribed for a specific individual, this is called a Patient-Specific Direction (PSD) and includes the dose, route and frequency or appliance to be supplied or administered to a named patient. These drugs are the property of the patient and to use it or them for someone else is theft. Nurses should therefore refer to DH (2006) *Medicines Matters: A Guide to Mechanisms for the Prescribing, Supply and Administration of Medicines*. PSDs might also include a group of named people for vaccination although it is more usual for a Patient Group Direction (PGD) although these might not be named individuals (such as drop in centres for the 'flu vaccine). Nurse associates cannot supply or administer a PGD.

The prescription form is a legal document and is classified as 'secure stationery'. Suitably qualified registered nurses can prescribe and are governed by The Medicinal Products: Prescription by Nurses Act 1992. The Misuse of Drugs Act 1971 has three classifications relating to drugs that are liable to abuse and misuse. Class 1 is opiates such as diamorphine, class 2 is the intermediate drugs such as Codeine and class 3 would include the least harmful drugs such as Zopiclone.

Safe storage

The *Safe and Secure Handling of Medicines: A Team Approach* (RPSGB, 2005) states that nurses must adhere to regulations for the proper storage of medicines, and all drugs should be stored within locked cupboards/drug trolleys/refrigerators. Controlled drugs should be in a locked cupboard, within a locked cupboard and these have a Controlled Drug Register which should be signed by at least one registered nurse and someone assessed as competent to sign the CDR; the CDR should similarly be kept in secure storage. In care settings, quite often the drug trolley is chained to a wall for added security.

When receiving drugs, it is important that they are properly checked in against the prescription to ensure the correct in date, drug, dose and route. This job should be performed by at least one registered nurse, in a safe environment without interruptions to prevent errors. Out of date drugs should be returned to the pharmacy for safe disposal and stock drugs should be rotated and checked regularly so administration errors do not occur.

Most drugs supplied to care settings come in pre-prepared dose formats. These are additionally regulated by The Health and Social Care Act 2008 (Regulated Activities) Regulations (2014), specifically 'Safe Care and Treatment' (Regulation 12) ensures the 'the proper and safe management of medicines'. Monitored Dosage Systems (MDS) are promoted as a safe system as it is clearly apparent when a drug has been removed from the packaging; however, it is not suitable for all drugs such as medicines that are susceptible to moisture, e.g. dispersible aspirin or light-sensitive medicines such as Chlorpromazine. Care settings who cannot afford the MDS system should not secondary dispense, i.e. decant drugs into compliance systems (such as Dosette boxes) (NHS Good Practice Guide, 2017). When the patient's own medicines are brought into a care setting, it is important to document the patient's consent to remote storage (in a suitable drugs storage facility). When administering the patient's own supply of drugs kept in their own room or locker, they should still be checked against the prescription and recorded as given on a Medication Administration Record (MARs) sheet or e-recording system. Many hospitals have adopted e-prescribing systems, the motivation being to improve the safety of medicines used and reduce the unacceptable levels of adverse drug events. According to Westbrook et al. (2009) a systematic review found a clear reduction in prescribing errors when e-prescribing was introduced.

Administration

Workers administering medication need to be accountable for their actions and should be assessed as competent to support the patient in taking medication. You should know the settings policies and procedures and understand that maladministration carries consequence for all. Before giving drugs, ensure that you have checked the items in the box below and you have washed your hands and are wearing personal protection.

> **Always check:** Patient's identity, any known allergies, check the drug matches the prescription (dose, format, delivery route), check the expiry date, do not give the medicine if an adverse reaction has occurred (you should contact the prescriber for advice and complete a yellow card), ensure the drug is administered at the correct time, record accurately if the medication has been taken (or refused).
>
> NB: If the patient has any cognitive deficiency, a current photograph and/or wristband is an acceptable alternative for identification.

Errors in administration need to be reported and recorded however, MHRA has reported its concerns that this does not happen often enough or in any meaningful way and suggest changes need to be made to the clinical governance of medication error reporting. They state: 'Incident reports are not always reviewed locally by staff with medication safety expertise to check quality and to initiate action before being submitted to the National Reporting and Learning Systems (NRLS)' (MHRA, 2017). Standard 24 of the NMC Standards for Medicines states: 'As a registrant, if you make an error you must take any action to prevent any potential harm to the patient and report as soon as possible to the prescriber, your line manager or employer (according to local policy) and document your actions. Midwives should also inform their named supervisor of midwives'. All errors are classed as 'patient safety incidents' and should be reported through local risk management systems. Management investigations are recommended to use the NPSA 'Being open' tool (saferhealthcare.org.uk) to reach disciplinary decisions when considering allegations of misconduct. Research by NPSA (2007) found that 7% of patients suffered harm by maladministration, mainly caused by interruptions while nurses were on the drug round. The box below details incident and frequency.

When patients are transferred from settings, for example from a care setting to a hospital, or between wards, NICE recommend that you accurately list all of the person's medicines (including prescribed, over-the-counter and complementary medicines) and carry out medicines reconciliation within 24 hours or sooner and that this should be recorded (online or paper based system).

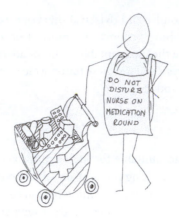

- Wrong dose, strength, frequency: 28.7%
- Omitted medicine: 17%
- Wrong medicine: 11.5%
- Wrong patient: 5%
- Patient allergic: 3.2%
- Wrong formulation: 2.4%
- Wrong route: 2.1%

Figure 7.7   Drug round

Right to Refuse

Patients have the right to refuse medication, and you must respect the patient's rights and record this to convention. It is importance to gain consent to treat from the patient as invasive devises such as drips and cannulas should not be interfered with (see above for rights of consent). Patients suffering poor mental health should be assessed using The Mental Capacity Act 2005 and in some instances, such as a Community Treatment Order (The Mental Health Act 1983, 2007) medication is enforced. Additionally, the GP may give consent for 'disguising' or covert medication if it is essential, this should be documented and advice sought from the pharmacist for the best means. NICE offer advice considering that 'If a patient is not taking their medicines, discuss with them whether this is because of beliefs and concerns or problems about the medicines (intentional non-adherence) or because of practical problems (unintentional non-adherence)' (NICE, 2017). Guidance should be given to the patient and a risk assessment should be included within the plan of care.

Adverse Drug Events

Adverse drug reactions (ADR) are an 'unwanted or harmful reaction experienced following the administration of a drug or combination of drugs under normal conditions of use' (NHS. gov, 2017), some side effects are known and documented, others maybe previously unrecognised. Detection and reporting is important as it is vital drugs are safe to use. Reporting systems are hosted by the MHRA through the 'yellow card' scheme which can be downloaded from the MHRA website (www.gov.uk/the-yellow-card-scheme-guidance-for-healthcare-professionals#how-to-report). Pharmacovigilance systems monitor drugs in everyday use.

Medically significant events are those that are fatal, life threatening, disabling, or lead to congenital abnormalities. An example of this is the repurposing of the drug Thalidomide intended for patients suffering leprosy or cancer (myeloma), it had a sedative effect and was thus marketed to pregnant women suffering hyperemesis (it was sold over-the counter in Europe). It caused congenital deformities such as malformation of the limbs (phocomelia) and organ deformities if taken in the first trimester. Drug companies have been fined and had their products removed from the market if they have been proven to cause serious side effects.

Unwanted side effects can act as a preventative to patient compliance, some are minor inconveniences for instance, diphenhydramine (Benadryl) eases allergy symptoms but it also suppresses acetylcholine which can lead to drowsiness and a dry mouth. Side effects also occur when patients mix drugs with alcohol (accidental overdose) or when the patient inadvertently takes too many of a drug (for example Warfarin dissolves blood clots but in overdose can cause internal bleeding). Drinking grapefruit juice when taking antihypertensive medication can affect its potency, as can mixing prescription medication with folk (herbal) remedies.

It is important to discuss any concerns with the patient so they can make an informed choice regarding their medication. It is remarkable how many patients leave the clinic or GP surgery with no clear idea of what drug they are taking or why and this lack of understanding leads to erratic or noncompliance in medication regimes.

Medication and the elderly

Older patients tend to suffer from impairment of function in the liver and kidneys (see Chapter 5), therefore important pharmacokinetic and pharmacodynamic changes occur in old age. A reduction in renal and hepatic function has pharmacokinetic consequence in terms of drug metabolism and clearance, leading to a longer drug half-life (such as digoxin), pharmacodynamic change might include increased sensitivity to drugs such as anticoagulants, cardiovascular and psychotropic drugs (Mangoni and Jackson, 2004). Ageing is associated with a reduction in first-pass metabolism, probably due to reduction of liver mass and reduced blood flow in the cardio compromised. Malnourished older patients (and those with protein deficiency disorders such as PEM) have reduced bioavailability for drugs such as Diazepam and Warfarin, also a reduction in renal function affects the clearance of many drugs such as water-soluble antibiotics and diuretics. Mangoni and Jackson (2004) consider that elderly patients 'are particularly vulnerable to adverse effects from neuroleptics' and can develop postural hypotension and cardiac arrhythmias as a result. The observant carer will note and report adverse effects to the prescriber.

Medical devices

Medical devises are regulated by The Medicines and Healthcare Products Regulatory Agency and Department of Health and are usefully defined by The World Health Organization (2017) as 'any instrument, apparatus, implement, machine, appliance, implant, reagent for in vitro use, software, material or other similar or related article, intended by the manufacturer to be used, alone or in combination, for human beings', and can be used for diagnosis, prevention, monitoring, treatment or alleviation of disease.

Medical technology is a rapidly developing arena, it is now common for cardiac function to be supported by implants which regulate and stimulate the heartbeat, to relive arthrosclerosis by stent, contraceptive implants, prosthetic blood vessels, hearing implants, renal dialysis and prosthetic limbs (to name but a few). It is not hard to imagine AI robotic surgery and artificial laboratory grown organs to replace worn out or diseased ones. Technology is used in the laboratory for diagnostic purposes, MRI/PET/CAT scanners are now in every major hospital (and shopping malls in America) making x-ray machines nearly redundant.

On wards, computers and tablets (such as iPads) are used for daily health recording and monitoring systems, patient records and drug management. Even before the patient arrives at A & E, paramedics will have used computerised systems to inform medical staff of the prospective patient's condition. You might have used computer software for training (such as safemedicate), and medical staff have used virtual reality devices for training surgeons. The current 'Transformation and sustainability' programme will promote remote/virtual GP appointments, with the patient wearing devices which record and transmit vital signs. However, protecting electronic data from 'hacking' or unethical use is a major issue.

The Data Protection Act was created to offer protection against misuse of personal information, the Department of Health hosts the Guidance for Reporting, Managing and Investigating Information Governance and Cyber Security Serious Incidents, with a digital helpdesk to report security breaches requiring investigation using an e-notification form. If you use an electronic device which stores patient data, it must be password protected and safely kept where it is not easily accessible for theft. Your employer will have e-safety protocols about information sharing and confidentiality, and you should familiarise yourself with them to protect your patients' data.

CHAPTER SUMMARY

- This chapter has introduced you to some basic maths used in healthcare. It has also discussed the importance of gaining consent prior to engaging in taking observations and shown you how to take the observations.
- You have also considered health and safety and the legislation that you need to be aware of when monitoring vital signs. This chapter has guided you to consider how to prepare yourself and your patient so that you are both safe and comfortable with the activity.
- You must ensure that you are properly trained and that you are judged competent by a professional assessor to engage in these activities before you undertake them with your patients.
- Medicines management considered the laws, policies and procedures for the safe administration and storage of medicines.

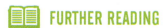 FURTHER READING

Websites

Researching these websites will enhance your understanding and deepen your knowledge of the issues covered in this chapter:

- Health data: https://ico.org.uk/for-organisations/health/
- Managing medicines in care homes: www.nice.org.uk/guidance/sc1
- Medical devices: www.gov.uk/topic/medicines-medical-devices-blood/medical-devices-regulation-safety
- Medicines optimisation guide: www.nice.org.uk/guidance/ng5
- MHRA (Medicines and Healthcare products Regulatory Agency): www.gov.uk/government/organisations/medicines-and-healthcare-products-regulatory-agency

- NEWS: www.rcplondon.ac.uk/projects/outputs/national-early-warning-score-news
- NMC (National Midwifery Council) Standards for Medicines Management: www.nmc.org.uk/standards/additional-standards/standards-for-medicines-management/
- Resuscitation Council lifesupport guidelines: www.resus.org.uk/resuscitation-guidelines/
- Secure and safe handling of medicines: a team approach: www.rpharms.com/making-a-difference/projects-and-campaigns/safe-and-secure-handling-of-medicines
- Wound management: dressing formulary: www.evidence.nhs.uk/formulary/bnf/current/a5-wound-management-products-and-elasticated-garments

Books

The following books will help you to deepen your understanding of essential skills:

- Delves-Yates, C. (2015) *Essential Clinical Skills for Nurses: Step by Step.* London: Sage.
- Starkings, S. (2015) *Passing Calculations Tests for Nursing Students* (Transforming Nursing Practice Series). London: Sage.
- Whelan, A. and Hughes, E. (2016) *Clinical Skills for Healthcare Assistants and Assistant Practitioners.* Chichester: Wiley.

Journal article

- Bennett, M.A. (1995) Report of the task force on the implications for darkly pigmented intact skin in the predication and prevention of pressure ulcers. *Advances in Wound Care*, 8(6): 34–5.

REFERENCES

Department of Health (2006) *Medicines Matters: A Guide to Mechanisms for the Prescribing, Supply and Administration of Medicines.* Available at: http://webarchive.nationalarchives.gov.uk/20130123191451/http://www.dh.gov.uk/en/Publicationsandstatistics/Publications/PublicationsPolicyAndGuidance/DH 064325 (accessed 4 July 2017).

Foucault, M. (1963) *The Birth of the Clinic: An Archaeology of Medical Perception.* London: Tavistock.

HSE (2016) *Infection in Care Homes.* Available at: www.hse.gov.uk/pbns/infection.pdf.

Mangoni, A. and Jackson, S. (2004) Age-related changes in pharmacokinetics and pharmacodynamics: basic principles and practical applications. *British Journal of Clinical Pharmacology.* 57(1): 6-14.

MHRA (2017) *Yellow Card.* Available at: https:/lvellowcard.mhra.gov.uk/(accessed 5 July 2017).

NICE (2017) *Medicines Management.* Available at: www.nice.org.uk/guidance/service-delivery--organisation-and-staffing/medicines-management (accessed 5 July 2017).

NPSA (2007) *Toolkits.* Available at: www.nrls.npsa.nhs.uk/resources/type/toolkits/ (accessed 5 July 2017).

RPSGB (200S)*Secure and Safe Handling of Medicines: A Team Approach.* Available at: www.rpharms.com/what-we-re-working-on/safe-and-secure-handling-of-medicines.asp (accessed 4 July 2017).

Westbrook, J., Reckman, M., Li, L., et al. (2012) Effects of two commercial electronic prescribing systems on prescribing error rates in hospital in-patients: a before and after study. *PLOS ONE.* Available at: www.ncbi.nlm.nih.gov/pubmed/22303286(accessed 5 July 2017).

World Health Organization (2017) *Medical Devices.* Available at: www.who.int/medical devices/en/ (accessed 5 July 2017).

8

APPLIED HEALTH SCIENCES

Gillian Rowe

This chapter will introduce you to the psychology and sociology of health, and it has content links with Chapter 12, Protecting Children and Vulnerable Adults. You will develop an understanding of psychological theory and sociological factors and how these can impact on an individual's health and life chances. The first part will focus on developing an understanding of underpinning psychological theories in relation to health and illness and will examine the role of psychology as an explanation of development through the life span. The second part will identify sociological theories and theorists that explain inequality in health and life chances.

Glossary

- **Attachment** The emotional relationship between a child and the established caregiver
- **Conditioning** The ways in which events, stimuli and behaviour become associated with one another
- **Hierarchy of needs** Maslow's view that human motives form a hierarchy from basic to complex
- **Nature–nurture debate** Discusses the relative importance of nature (heritable) and experience (nurture) in determining development and behaviour

INTRODUCTION

This chapter is intended to equip you with an understanding of the psychology of health and illness and how sociological factors impact on the health of an individual, family and society. Every human being is different. We all grow and change over time physically, mentally, emotionally and socially. So, what makes us who we are and what determines what sort of person we become? What determines the lives we lead? Think about Table 8.1, and consider what has determined who you are.

Table 8.1 Nature or nurture? What determines who we are – genetics or the environment we are born into?

Nature	Nurture
We all agree we inherited our physical characteristics from our parents – but did we also inherit our behaviour and personality?	Refers to environmental influences. This can include any factors from before, during and after birth as well as factors during our upbringing such as nutrition, cultural expectations, education, family

DEVELOPMENT ACROSS THE LIFE SPAN

The arguments

Some theorists think that development occurs continuously where individuals gradually add more of the same type of skills. Others argue that development takes place discontinuously as individuals change rapidly with new understanding at specific times. Figure 8.1 demonstrates this.

In order to understand psychological theory, this part of the chapter is grouped by psychological themes to give you a basic understanding of who the theorist is and how their theory fits within the main paradigms. Psychology for health is a relatively new branch of psychology and this means new interpretations of established

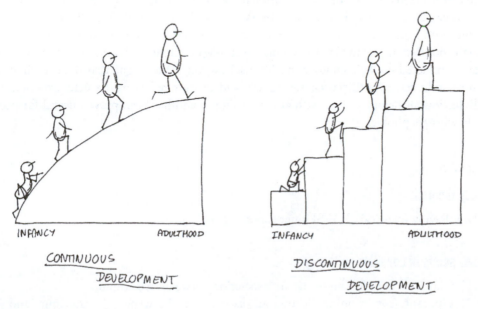

INFANCY   ADULTHOOD   INFANCY   ADULTHOOD

CONTINUOUS   DISCONTINUOUS
  DEVELOPMENT   DEVELOPMENT

Figure 8.1 Theories of development

theory. The interaction between the mind and body, a person's health beliefs and coping mechanisms, all contribute to the success (or otherwise) of an intervention and recovery. Research (Doll and Peto, 1981; Blot and Tarone, 2015) has shown that health behaviours have a contributing effect on the likelihood of developing cancer. Smoking tobacco causes 30% of all lung cancers and poor diet is responsible for 35% of other cancers (such as bowel cancer). Therefore, if someone's coping mechanism for psychological stress is to smoke and eat junk food, there is a statistical probability of them developing cancer. Heart disease can develop as a result of high cholesterol in the cardiovascular system, the burden of overnutrition being a leading contributory source. As one eminent cardiac surgeon said, 'the chance of developing heart disease is 50% genes and 50% burger'.

Behaviourism

Key theorists

John B. Watson, Ivan Pavlov, Burrhus Frederic Skinner, Albert Bandura, Edward Thorndike

Key points of behaviourist theory

This theory posits the notion that we are born as a clean slate (*tabula rasa*) and that there is no such thing as free will, as all behaviour is learned from our environment as a response to stimulus and therefore it is considered deterministic. Theorists believe that this mechanism is common to animals and that the behaviour of humans and animals can be compared. Experiments by Watson and Rayner (1920) on 'Little Albert' to condition him to be frightened of rats were successful and prompted further research. Behaviourists are credited with making psychology a scientific discipline as experiments are conducted under laboratory conditions; however, critics argue that the experiments are conducted in artificial circumstances and do not reflect 'real world' experiences. Behavioural therapy is used with autistic children and has been proven useful for people who are phobic.

Conditioning

Key theorists

Ivan Pavlov (classical), B.F. Skinner (operant)

Key points of conditioning theory

[1] Classical conditioning forms an association between two stimuli.
[2] Operant conditioning forms an association between a behaviour and a consequence.

There are four possible consequences to any behaviour. They are:

a. Something Good can start or be presented
b. Something Good can end or be taken away
c. Something Bad can start or be presented
d. Something Bad can end or be taken away

Psychodynamic theory

Key theorists

Sigmund Freud, Erik Erikson

Key points of the psychodynamic approach

We move through a series of stages during our life span in which there is an apparent conflict between biological drives and social expectations. The way in which this conflict is resolved is the main determining factor in our ability to learn, get along with others and cope with anxiety. There is a presumption that unconscious forces of which we are unaware manifest themselves in the things we say and do. The psychodynamic approach conflicts with Behaviourism by suggesting that behaviour and feelings are affected by unconscious motives and that all behaviour has an unconscious cause. This has a relationship with our upbringing and may have been laid down before we were able to speak. Freud is considered as the 'father of psychology' although it could be argued that Charles Darwin first described adaptive behaviours in his work on evolution. Table 8.2 explains Freud's theory of personality and Table 8.3 lists the stages of development and complexes.

Freud considers that the ego operates mainly in conscious and preconscious levels, although it also contains elements of the unconscious because both the Ego and the Super Ego evolved from the Id. Figure 8.2 encapsulates the theory.

Freud's stages of development

- Oral stage
- Anal stage
- Phallic stage

Table 8.2 Freud's theory of personality: *The Ego and the Id* (2010 [1923])

The Super Ego	The set of moral controls given to us by outside influences. It is our moral code or conscience and is often in conflict with the Id
The Ego	The conscious self, the part seen by the outside world
The Id	The unconscious self, the part of the mind containing basic drives and repressed memories. It is amoral, has no concern about right and wrong and is only concerned with itself

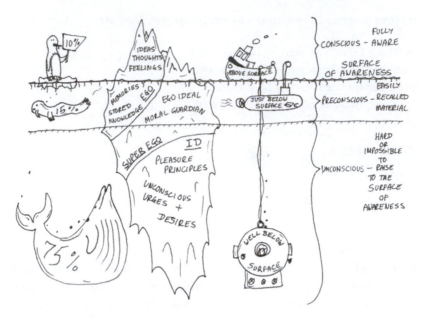

Figure 8.2   Freud's iceberg theory

In order to develop psychologically, the child must resolve the Oedipus/Electra conflict:

> Oedipus complex = male child's desire for sexual involvement with his mother
>
> Electra complex = female child's desire for sexual involvement with father

Freud considers that both lead to a deep-seated feeling of guilt starting at a very young age. Erik Erikson (1994 [1959]) took Freud's idea's further. He believed that the ego developed through a set of stages, at the end of which there was a crisis which needed to be resolved for the individual to move onto the next stage. Erikson's stages (Table 8.3) argue that psychological maturity depends on how well the conflict is resolved.

Table 8.3   Erikson's stages

Infant: Basic Trust vs. Mistrust: responsive care vs. neglect

Toddler: Autonomy vs. Shame: independence vs. forced action

Preschool: Initiative vs. Guilt: initiative vs. control

School-age Child: Industry vs. Inferiority: sense of self vs. bullying

Freud's theories of development ended at adolescence; however, Erikson considered that there are eight life stages

Adolescent: Identity vs. role confusion: self-identity Vs. no clear identity

Young Adult: Intimacy vs. Isolation: meaningful relationships Vs. self-isolation

Middle-aged Adult: Generativity vs. Self-absorption: having children and productive work vs. selfishness

Older Adult: Integrity vs. Despair: life accomplishment vs. life dissatisfaction

Critics of Erikson's stages point out that this is a very Western-centric viewpoint that does not translate globally and that it is misogynistic as it does not take women's life experiences into account.

 Scenario 8.1

You are supporting adults with mental health problems in a group home in the community. One group member (Amy) comes in to your office, she is very upset as she has spent all her weekly cash allowance and has no money left to buy food. You give her sympathy and a cup of tea and then offer some money to help her out for the rest of the week.

Amy is relieved and grateful but – what has Amy learned from this? What are the drawbacks of this from a behavioural perspective? What might have been a better response?

The cognitive approach

Key theorists

Jean Piaget, Edward Tolman

Key points of the cognitive approach

The cognitive approach conflicts with behaviourist theory as it focuses on internal processes rather than external behaviour. Cognitivism sometimes makes comparisons between humans and computers processing information. It considers that behaviour can be largely explained in terms of how the mind operates, that is, the information processing approach. Piaget stated in *The Construction of Reality in the Child* (1954) that he believed intelligence is fixed at birth and that children actively seek to understand the world they live in. He believed they learn through experience and developed what he called 'schemas' to make sense of the world around them.

Piaget believed that children pass through four stages of cognitive development (Table 8.4).

Tolman (1948) cited by Hothersall (2003) believed individuals do more than merely respond to stimuli, that they act on beliefs, attitudes, changing conditions, and they strive toward goals. Tolman is virtually the only behaviourist who found the stimulus–response theory unacceptable; because reinforcement was not necessary for learning to occur, he felt behaviour was mainly cognitive.

Social learning theory

Key theorists

Albert Bandura, Lev Vygotsky, Jean Lave

Table 8.4   Piaget's theory of cognitive development

Birth to 2 years	Sensorimotor stage: children learn assimilation and accommodation
Ages 2 to 4	Preoperational stage: not able to abstractly conceptualise, needs concrete objects
Ages 7 to 11	Concrete operations: able to abstractly conceptualise
Ages 11 to 15	Formal operations: capable of deductive and hypothetical reasoning

Key points of social learning theory

Social learning theory is considered a bridge between behavioural and cognitive theory. Bandura (1977) considered that children learn through modelling 'significant others' behaviours. He used the 'Bobo doll experiment' (1961–63) to prove this. This theory examines how social influences, personal factors and behaviours interact. The theory explains how we might choose to adopt the behaviours of a role model. Bandura went on to develop the theory of 'Social Cognitive Learning' (1986), which is called triangulate reciprocal determinism: behaviour, personal factors and environment. Self-efficacy is a core factor in the triangulate mechanism. Self-efficacy is about self-appraisal and self-belief, and this influences beliefs about what a person can (or cannot) achieve (Figure 8.3).

Humanism

Key theorists

Carl Rogers, Abraham Maslow

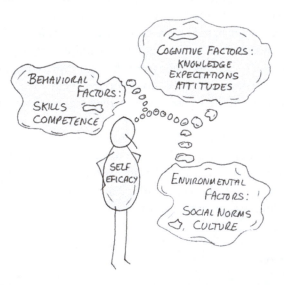

Figure 8.3   Self-efficacy

Key points of the humanistic approach

Humanism studies the whole person; therefore, it is considered holistic. The theory states that behaviour is connected to feelings and self-concept. A humanist looks at behaviours through the eyes of the individual doing the behaviour to understand their motives and drives. Humanism rejects behaviourism as it considers the theory to be deterministic and mechanistic. Humanists also consider it lacks understanding regarding promoting personal agency as it does not acknowledge free will. Both Rogers and Maslow believed that people could overcome adversity and achieve fulfilment and satisfaction, which was named 'self-actualisation'. Humanism also rejects the scientific method and promotes qualitative methods such as writing reflective journals based on thinking and feeling. When constructing the hierarchy of needs (1943), Maslow studied those he believed were successful and productive. Kenrick et al. (2010) consider the hierarchy pyramid to be 'one of the most cognitively contagious ideas in the behavioural sciences'. Maslow determined that once one need was satisfied, a person could then move up the pyramid. It should be stated that everyone has their own personal take on the pyramid, an idea of what constitutes *for them* notions of achieving each level, and each person will have a different view of what self-actualisation means. Activity 8.1 offers you the chance to think about some of the criticism of hierarchy.

 Activity 8.1

Do you agree with the pyramid? Although used by feminist Betty Friedan in *The Feminine Mystique* (1963), other critics have said that this is a male pyramid. Cullen (1974) considers the hierarchy 'misinterpreted women's experience and sexuality, and valued only those women with stereotypically masculine characteristics and behaviours'. Other critics, such as Neher (1991), have also said that the pyramid is Western ethnocentric and its concepts and language do not apply to other cultures.

Reflect on the concepts contained in the pyramid and consider whose account you would agree with.

Carl Rogers believed that every person can achieve their goals, wishes and desires in life. He said that how we think about ourselves, our feelings of self-worth, are of fundamental importance both to psychological health and to the likelihood that we can achieve goals and ambitions in life. He said 'This process of the good life is not, I am convinced, a life for the faint-hearted. It involves the stretching and growing of becoming more and more of one's potentialities. It involves the courage to be. It means launching oneself fully into the stream of life' (Rogers, 1961).

Attachment theory

See also Chapter 12, Protecting Children and Vulnerable Adults, which gives more detail on attachment theory.

Key theorists

John Bowlby, Mary Ainsworth, Cindy Hazan, Philip Shaver

Key points of attachment theory

Attachment theory is based on the idea that our first relationship with our primary carer (usually the mother) shapes the way we relate to others throughout our lives. It covers two important aspects of attachment formation and although it is a single theory, it is convenient to look at it in two parts:

[1] The way in which children form attachment bonds and the nature of these bonds.
[2] What happens if these bonds are not formed properly, i.e., the effects of deprivation and privation has on a child.

Children have an instinctive need to attach to one person and are biologically 'pre-programmed' to make such an attachment; the attachment process keeps the child safe. There is a critical period, from 7 months to 3 years, during which the baby is most likely to form this attachment bond. If it is not formed by the age of about 3, it is unlikely to form at all and the child may never attach to anyone. This can have a considerable impact on the ability to form successful relationships in later life. The main characteristics of attachment are shown in Table 8.5. Schaffer (1996) described attachment as 'A long-enduring, emotionally meaningful tie to a particular individual'.

Table 8.5   The characteristics of attachment

Attachments are selective - they are directed towards specific individuals who are preferred above all others
They involve the desire to be near the person they are attached to
They provide comfort and security and are particularly important when the child is upset, ill, or tired
They involve separation protest - the child becomes upset if they are separated from the person to whom they are attached

Signs of attachment

- Separation protest: Becomes distressed if their primary caregiver leaves the room and they cannot see her/him. They will cry and, if they are mobile, will crawl towards the door through which she/he left.

- Stranger anxiety: Very wary of strangers. If a stranger tries to interact with them while they are with their primary carer, they will ignore them or look away. If they are approached by a stranger when they are within the vicinity of the primary carer, they will move towards her/him quickly. If they are unable to crawl, they will put out their hands for her/him. Mary Ainsworth used the 'Strange situation experiment' to determine five types of attachment, which are detailed in Chapter 12.

Fraley and Shaver (2000) researched adult relationships and found that there is a correlation between childhood attachment types and romantic relationships in serving attachment-related functions; however, this research is considered incomplete.

Bowlby's maternal deprivation hypothesis (1953)

Children have an innate need for warm, continuous relationship. If the main bond is broken in early years, this will have adverse effects on emotional, social and cognitive development. This will impact on the ability to form relationships with others, the ability to form attachments, the ability to learn and upon language acquisition. Table 8.6 explains how maternal deprivation can affect the child's physical and mental development.

Table 8.6   Bowlby's research on the effects of maternal deprivation

Bed wetting (enuresis)

Physical underdevelopment (deprivation dwarfism)

Depression

Intellectual retardation

Inability to make relationships, affectionless psychopathy

 Scenario 8.2

Harry has been fostered by his relatives since his parents died when he was 12 months old. His relatives did not care for him properly because they considered him weird, and the relationship is fractured. At age 11, he chooses to leave this home and go to boarding school. At boarding school, Harry has only two friends, who are also considered odd. As he grows older, he develops a crush on another student, but Harry is incapable of dealing with his emotions and does nothing. The girl eventually pushes herself on him but to no avail. Harry always returns to the refuge that is his two friends. He rejects anyone who tries to become involved with him and he persists in trying to do everything by himself.

- How would you describe Harry in relation to the theorists you have learned about?
- Which theory best describes Harry's behaviour?

The life course perspective

The life course perspective recognises the importance of timing in lives, not just in terms of chronological age, but also in terms of biological age, psychological age, social age and spiritual age. This perspective emphasises the ways in which humans are interdependent and gives special attention to the family as the primary arena for experiencing and interpreting the wider social world, and recognises the linkages between childhood, adolescence and older age.

Families have an impact on the growing individual and the types of parenting style will influence the child's understanding of the world and the type of parent the child becomes. Diana Baumrind (1971) created a typology of parenting styles which offered three types of parenting – authoritarian, permissive and authoritative – which are considered archetypes of parenting. As a child ages, they start to form more complex friendships and peer relationships. It becomes emotionally important to have friends, especially of the same sex. They might also experience more peer pressure and begin to adopt non-family role models.

The child becomes more aware of his or her body as puberty approaches and eating problems sometimes start around this age. Adolescence marks the period of physical maturity, with important biological and sexual changes occurring. Adolescence is sometimes referred to as a period of 'storm and stress' as the child develops an independent attitude to school, the family and their environment. As children become adults they must deal psychologically, physically and emotionally with each transition.

⚙️ Activity 8.2

Look again at Erikson's theory of life span development in terms of the adolescent identity crisis and the struggle to establish a personal identity, or self-concept, and consider this in association with Bandura's social cognitive theory and self-efficacy beliefs.

Erikson says regarding the 'intimacy and isolation' stage, that it is the time 'to lose and find oneself in another – the giving and receiving of physical and emotional connection, support, love, comfort, trust and all the other elements that we would typically associate with healthy adult relationships conducive to mating and child-rearing'. He also says it could be a time of isolation and of being excluded.

How do you think this relates to the case study about Harry?

[Erikson himself struggled with his own identity after discovering that his stepfather was not his biological father. He had been bullied at his Jewish temple for not looking 'Jewish' as he was blond and blue-eyed. He dropped out of his studies and went travelling, eventually working with Anna Freud. When he emigrated to America in 1933, he changed his name from Homberger to 'Erikson', as he felt he was his own creation.]

Adult ageing was considered by Daniel Levinson (1986), who developed a 'seasons of life' model of development as a different explanation to Erikson, although it is still a stage model. All stage models (see Figure 8.4) are open to the criticism that they do not apply to all people everywhere.

These theories have a relationship with George Vaillant's (2002) 'Adult Tasks' theory and Bernice Neugarten's (1974) 'Social Clock' theory. The midlife crisis is considered a

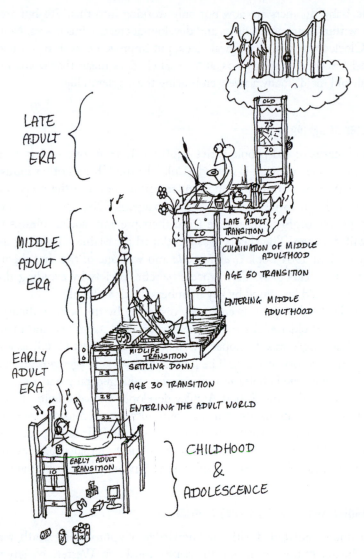

LATE ADULT ERA

MIDDLE ADULT ERA

EARLY ADULT ERA

OLD
75
70
65

LATE ADULT TRANSITION
CULMINATION OF MIDDLE ADULTHOOD
AGE 50 TRANSITION
ENTERING MIDDLE ADULTHOOD

60
55
50
45

MIDLIFE TRANSITION
SETTLING DOWN
AGE 30 TRANSITION
ENTERING THE ADULT WORLD

40
33
28
22

EARLY ADULT TRANSITION

17
10
4

CHILDHOOD & ADOLESCENCE

Figure 8.4   The stage model of development

time of revaluation that leads to questioning long-held beliefs and values. This may be the result of factors such as divorce, change in jobs, moving home, loss of parents/caring for parents. Typically beginning in the mid-40s, the crisis often occurs in response to a sense of mortality, as middle adults realise that their youth is limited and that they have not accomplished all of their desired goals in life. Not everyone experiences stress or upset during middle age, other middle-age adults prefer to reframe their experience by thinking of themselves as being in the prime of their lives rather than in their declining years, especially now that longevity has increased in the Western world. As the population ages, an interesting phenomenon is appearing, namely the migration of the age at which someone is considered old. People were considered officially old when they reached retirement age, however the Baby Boomers are now not only working into their 70s but are becoming more active within their communities and developing creative businesses. Neugarten tied the Social Clock to women's biological clock, but improvements in reproductive science has extended the child-bearing years, and social changes mean that women do not fear becoming an 'old maid', many actively embracing the singleton life.

Other theories of ageing

The role and status of old people varies enormously from one society to another, as does the age at which a person is viewed as 'old'. In the UK and other industrial countries, retirement from work is an important transition point in the process of growing old. Two conflicting theories explain attitudes to ageing. Disengagement theory argues that elderly people begin to disengage from their previous social roles as they realise that they will die soon. The theory was developed by Elaine Cumming and Warren Earl Henry in their 1961 book *Growing Old* and was one of the first theories of ageing developed by sociologists. This process benefits society by avoiding the potential disruption that would be caused by key members dying suddenly.

Subsequently, the theory has been largely disproven by the 'activity theory of ageing', which proposes that older adults are happiest when they stay active and maintain social interactions. The theory was developed by Robert J. Havighurst (1963) as a response to the disengagement theory of ageing. The process of successful ageing is greatly facilitated when older people pursue hobbies and relationships and generally lead a more active lifestyle. George L. Maddox and Robert Atchley developed the 'continuity theory' (Atchley, 1989), which considers internal structures of continuity remain constant over a lifetime and include elements such as personality traits, ideas and beliefs. It helps people make future decisions by providing them with a stable foundation. External structures of continuity help maintain a stable self-concept and lifestyle and include relationships and social roles.

Elisabeth Kübler-Ross and the stages of grief

When someone is confronted with the knowledge of approaching death, reactions can depend on the age of the person and the reason for death. Western society tends to be 'death denying', and often, reluctant to acknowledge someone is dying, important conversations are not said, or said too late.

The dying person may visit the stages before death, and after the death their family may also experience the stages while mourning their loss. Elisabeth Kübler-Ross (1969) proposed five stages in approaching death (Table 8.7), although not everyone follows the sequence through the stages and not all people experience all the stages. Grieving is a process and each person will experience it differently; there is no set time for visiting each stage and many return to some stages during the mourning process.

There are criticisms of Kübler-Ross' stage theory. Kastenbaum and Costa (1977) deny any evidence that the stages exist and suggest her data-gathering methodology is flawed, and Corr et al. (2007) considered the stages reductionist and therefore unhelpful as it rejects the person's ability to empower their own coping strategies.

Table 8.7   Kübler-Ross' stages of approaching death

Denial ('It must be a mistake')
Anger ('It isn't fair!')
Bargaining ('Let me/them live longer and I'll be a better person')
Depression ('I've lost everything important to me')
Acceptance ('What has to be, has to be')

WHAT IS PSYCHOLOGY FOR HEALTH?

Health psychology, often synonymous with behavioural medicine and medical psychology, is the application of psychological theory and research to health, illness and healthcare. Clinical psychology focuses on mental health and neurological illness; health psychology is concerned with the psychology of a range of health-related behaviour. Understanding psychological theory supports the care practitioner to understand the patient/client and make choices regarding interventions. Table 8.8 looks at the approaches you have examined in relation to psychology for health.

Table 8.8   Psychology for health

Psychological theory provides the basis of psychological approaches for intervention
The **behavioural** approach looks at observed behaviour
The **cognitive** approach listens to the client
The **humanistic** approach listens to the client and gives the client choices
The **psychodynamic** approach interprets what the person says and does

   The biopsychosocial model of health was developed by George Engel (1977) as a means to move the stale medical vs. social model of health debate forward (see Chapter 11 on mental health and wellbeing for further detail on the models of health). The biopsychosocial theory posits that each one of these factors is not sufficient to bring about health or psychological illness, but the interaction between them determines the course of one's development. The biological influences on mental health and mental illness are varied, and include genetics, infections, physical trauma, nutrition, hormones and toxins. The psychological component looks for potential psychological causes for a health problem, such as lack of self-control, emotional turmoil and negative thinking.
   Social and cultural factors are conceptualised as a set of stressful events (e.g., losing one's job) that can differentially impact mental health depending on the individual and the social context in which they live. Despite its usefulness, there are issues with the biopsychosocial model including the degree of influence that each factor has, the degree of interaction between factors, and variation across individuals and life spans.
   The biopsychosocial model states that the workings of both the body and the environment affect the mind, and the workings of the mind can affect the body and

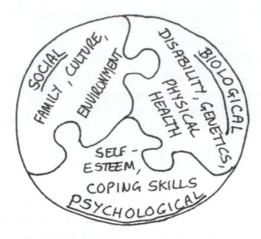

Figure 8.5   The biopsychosocial model

environment (see Figure 8.5). The theory posits that each one of these factors is not sufficient to bring about health or illness, but the interaction between them is what determines health outcomes

UNDERSTANDING AND EXPLAINING SOCIAL PHENOMENA

The Oxford English Dictionary states that 'Sociology is the scientific or academic study of social behaviour, including its origins, development, organisation, and institutions'. It is a social science that uses various methods of empirical investigation and critical analysis to develop a body of knowledge about social order, social disorder and social change. The origins of sociology lie in the nineteenth century when advances during 'The Enlightenment' led people to believe there was a rational explanation to the problems facing society. Auguste Comte (1798–1857) coined the name 'sociology', the science of society: ideas about society are conceptual, and research and evidence then lead to theoretical development, which is why it is a science.

Stated basically, the medical model assumes that the body is a machine that breaks down now and then and it is the role of medicine to repair it, reducing the role of medical and nursing staff to that of mechanic and technician. The social model examines the world that the body exists in and social science seeks to understand how culture, experience and society explains health and illness.

 Glossary

- **Constructivism** Knowledge is socially constructed on a shared understanding that forms the basis of an assumed reality (such as interactionism)

- **Empirical** Based on or verifiable by experience or observation
- **Iatrogenic** Ill health caused through medical intervention
- **Paradigm** A standard perspective or set of ideas
- **Pathogenic** Disease causing
- **Positivism** Scientific approach to gathering knowledge (such as functionalism)

What are paradigms?

Paradigms are used to explain ideas, rather like looking at something through a particular lens or perspective. Paradigms are broad perspectives or viewpoints that allow social scientists to have a variety of tools to describe the behaviour of the society, and be able to create hypothesis and theories. The notion of paradigms was developed by Thomas Kuhn (1962) to explain a set of changing circumstances or changes in knowledge resulting in changing circumstances.

Paradigms in sociology

Sociology has many perspectives, but this chapter will focus on three major paradigms and will apply them to the sociological enquiry into health.

The conflict paradigm

Key theorists

Karl Marx, Fredrick Engels, Ivan Illich

Key points of social conflict theory

Key elements in this perspective are that society is structured in ways to benefit a few at the expense of the majority, and factors such as wealth, property, race, sex, gender, class and age are linked to social inequality. To a social conflict theorist, this is all about dominant group versus minority group relations. Conflict is considered an engine for change to challenge an unequal social order and bring about equilibrium in resources and power.

Feminist theorists such as Abbot and Wallace (1990), Rege (2003) and Millett (2000) argue that none of the perspectives consider the roles and voice of women and they critique systems designed by and for (mainly white, middle class) men. Feminists focus on gender, disadvantage and health. The feminist perspective considers that health is paternalistic, especially in relation to the physiology of reproduction. Black women activists such as bel hooks (2001) call this 'intersectionality', where wealth, power and white privilege meet together to form an oppressive exclusive social system.

Conflict theory and health

This theory argues that people from disadvantaged social backgrounds are more likely to become ill and to receive inadequate healthcare. Dr Paul Farmer (1999) said that 'Inequality itself constitutes our modern plague – inequality is a pathogenic force'. Ivan Illich (1976) considered that medicine itself could be a force for ill and developed the theory of medical iatrogenesis. He considered this to take three forms (Table 8.9).

Table 8.9   Illich's three forms of medical iatrogenesis

Clinical	Social	Cultural
The damage done to patients through ineffective, unsafe and flawed treatments. He recommended that all treatments should be proven using evidence-based medicine. It could be argued that adverse psychological treatments and therapies comes under this heading	The medicalisation of social conditions such as sadness, age-related declines	Removing from people the ability to trust their own instincts regarding their health, and the ridicule of traditional ways of dealing with, and making sense of, death, suffering, and sickness. This reduces or encourages people to lose their autonomous coping skills. This might include homely remedies such as wearing a copper bracelet to ward off joint pain or using lay knowledge such as that described by Stacy (1994: 106): 'Not taking your child to the cold draughty health clinic on a pouring wet winter day is health giving rather than health denying, that's the intelligent use of lay knowledge'

Conflict theory considers that health should be a natural right and such things that promote health (safe employment, dry home, decent food, access to clean water, access to healthcare etc.) are human rights and not commodities only available to those who can afford them.

The functionalist paradigm (the positivist approach)

Key theorists

Auguste Compte, Emile Durkheim, Talcott Parsons

Key points of functionalism

Society consists of a system of interdependent institutions and organisations held together by shared values, common symbols (family, education, economy, polity and religion) that function for the survival of the society and functionalism is always oriented toward what is good for the whole of society. Functionalism considers society at the macro level and examines its core institutions and how they promote stability and productivity. Critics (such as Gramsci) consider that this stability is at the cost of progress and change, and calls this 'cultural hegemony' (Ayers, 2008).

Functionalism and health

Parsons considered that shared values led to common expectations, thus the individual replicates the norms of the society she/he has lived in, and this is considered to underpin socialisation and social control. Socialisation is supported by the positive and negative sanctioning of role behaviours that do or do not meet these expectations. Parsons (1951) considered that ill health is a social phenomenon or 'an unmotivated deviance' rather than a physical/mental disorder, stating that health is 'The state of optimum capacity of an individual for the effective performance of the roles and tasks for which s/he has been socialised.'

Parsons (1951) considered 'the sick role' and explained that in order to meet society's expectations, the sick person needed to perform functions within the sick role and therefore had certain rights and obligations (see Table 8.10 for an explanation of the sick role), and in the process makes doctors agents of social control, for instance by writing sick notes to allow time off work to be ill.

Table 8.10   The obligations of the sick role

Rights	Obligations
1. The sick person is exempt from 'normal' social roles relative to the nature and severity of the illness	The sick person should try to get well. The first two aspects of the sick role are conditional upon the third aspect
2. The sick person is not responsible for his or her condition, an individual's illness is usually thought to be beyond his or her own control	The sick person should seek technically competent help, and cooperate with the physician
A morbid condition of the body needs to be changed and some curative process apart from person's will power or motivation is needed to get well	

If the sick person does not comply with the strictures of the role, then they are said to be 'malingering', and therefore are not deserving of our sympathy. This has implications for people suffering from the side effects of drugs; if they stop taking them they are labelled 'non-compliant' and therefore undeserving of further help.

The symbolic interactionist paradigm

Key theorists

George Herbert Mead, Charles Horton Cooley, Howard Becker, Ervine Goffman, Émile Durkheim

Key points of the interactionist paradigm

This paradigm considers that reality is socially constructed through our interactions with one another. Morality, ethics and values are not a given; we create them through our interactions with one another. Therefore, it must follow that health and ill health must be social constructs and that society determines them. Social action is influenced by a person's beliefs, attitudes, perceptions and negotiations of meanings. Language plays a role in the interactions, and individuals are called 'social actors'. Through interaction we act out the roles that make up our day-to-day life. Mead (1934) separates the 'I' and 'Me' (Figure 8.6) in his 'theory of the social self' in our interactions, and these make up our concept of self and are situated within a social context. Scenario 8.3 explains this concept.

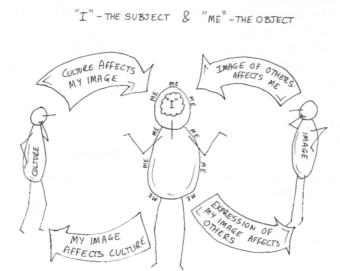

Figure 8.6   Mead's I and me

💬 Scenario 8.3

You have tripped and fallen over and the pain in your knee makes you want to cry ('I'). However (the social context), you do not want to look like a wimp in front of your friends ('Me'), so you just swear instead (social context) or laugh it off if swearing is unacceptable.

Howard Becker (1963) said that society creates rules, and by doing this anyone who acts outside of these rules is a deviant. This has a relationship with labelling theory (Becker, Goffman). Durkheim (1951 [1897]) explains that society's attitude will label some behaviours as deviant, such as 'committing' suicide. Social stigma labels the families of social deviants (criminals, gays, transgender, mentally ill) as part of that deviancy. Once someone has been labelled as deviant, it is hard to escape the role society has created for you. Goffman (1963) calls this role 'the resident alien'. Cooley (1930 [1902]) examined self-image and said we see ourselves through the eyes of other people, and that we incorporate their views of us into our own self-concept. He said this is made of three components (see Table 8.11) and this can lead to self-doubt and feelings of insecurity. Cooley determined that our self-view is a reflection of how others see us.

Table 8.11   Cooley's three components

We imagine how we must appear to others.

We imagine and react to what we feel their judgement of that appearance must be

We develop our self through the judgements of others

Source: Yeung and Martin, 2003

Go Further 8.1

'The Looking Glass Self' – watch the video from the Khan Academy on YouTube: www.youtube.com/watch?v=bU0BQUa11ek

---

SYMBOLIC INTERACTIONISM AND HEALTH

These theorists consider that health and ill health are social constructs. Interactionists look for the meaning within these terms and consider that ill health is a form of deviance (somewhat as Parsons considered). However, if you change the word 'bad' into 'sick', you can create a new meaning and 'normalise' unacceptable behaviours. For instance, alcoholics were once considered the dregs of society, but now that alcoholism is understood to be a disease, it is not so stigmatised. Mental health however, is still stigmatised. Activity 8.3 looks at stigma and Anglo-Caribbean men.

Activity 8.3

Black Anglo-Caribbean men make up 2% (2011 Census data) of the population but black people are three times more likely to be admitted to psychiatric hospitals in England and Wales and black people are up to 44% more likely to be detained under the Mental Health Act. Within psychiatric services, black men are about 50% more likely than average to be put into seclusion in closed rooms (figures from 'Count Me In' mental health and ethnicity census, 2005). The last 'Count me in' was undertaken in 2011, and very little has changed over the years; black men are still overrepresented in rates of detention under the Mental Health Act and have higher rates of seclusion (confinement in a locked room) than other groups by ethnicity (CQC, 2011).

Why do you think young black men are overrepresented within mental health services? Use symbolic interactive theory to offer an explanation.

As Britain is a multicultural society, we need to think about cultural differences in social meanings of illness and healthcare delivery. Not giving sufficient consideration to cultural beliefs and needs can lead to isolation of ethnic groups and misunderstandings about healthcare needs. Marginalising ethnic groups can lead to false health assumptions, such as for Black Anglo-Caribbean men, and lead to poor health for women and children, especially maternity services and post-natal care.

CHAPTER SUMMARY

- This chapter has given you an introduction to the sociology of health. You have gained an understanding that health and disease are essentially contested (this means there is no one single agreement on what this means).
- Sickness is only legitimate if a medical practitioner says it is, and ailments can receive or lose legitimacy (homosexuality was once classed as a disease, alcoholism was once classed as a moral failing). Therefore, notions of disease and sickness are culturally mediated. How we understand ourselves and our roles in health depends on the lens or perspective we use to view this phenomenon.
- By gaining an understanding of your patients' lives, their psychological roots and their social backgrounds, you will also have a better understanding of how people behave and react as they do when they come into contact with the caring services and how they cope with illness, pain and the demands of everyday life.

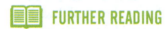 FURTHER READING

These texts will help you to develop your understanding of the psychology and sociology of health and the websites will give you up-to-date insights. You can watch videos about all the theoretical perspectives on YouTube.

Websites

- The SocioWeb: www.socioweb.com
- UK Data Archive: www.data-archive.ac.uk
- British Sociological Association: www.britsoc.co.uk
- Office for National Statistics: http://ons.gov.uk/ons/taxonomy/index.html?nscl=Health+and+Social+Care

Books

- Beckett, C. and Taylor, H. (2012) *Human Growth and Development*. London: Sage.
- Crawford, K. (2010) *Social Work and Human Development* (3rd edn). London: Sage.
- Giddens, A. and Sutton, P. (2013) *Sociology* (7th edn). Cambridge: Polity Press.
- Gleitman, H., Gross, J. and Reisberg, D. (2007) *Psychology* (7th edn). London: Norton.
- Illich, I. (1976) *Limits to Medicine: Medical Nemesis – The Expropriation of Health*. London: Boyers Publishing.
- Nettleton, S. (2013) *The Sociology of Health and Illness* (3rd edn). Cambridge: Polity Press.
- Sudbury, J. (2009) *Human Growth and Development*. London: Routledge.

REFERENCES

Abbott, P. and Wallace, C. (1990) *An Introduction to Sociology: Feminist Perspectives*. London: Routledge.

Atchley, R.C. (1989) A continuity theory of normal aging. *The Gerontologist*, 29(2): 183–90.

Ayers, A. (2008) *Gramsci, Political Economy, and International Relations Theory*. Basingstoke: Palgrave Macmillan.

Bandura, A. (1977) *Social Learning Theory* (Prentice-Hall Series in Social Learning). Englewood Cliffs, NJ: Prentice–Hall.

Bandura, A. (1986) *Social Foundations of Thought and Action: A Social Cognitive Theory*. Englewood Cliffs, NJ: Prentice–Hall.

Baumrind, D. (1971) Current patterns of parental authority (Developmental Psychology Monograph). *Developmental Psychology*, 4(1, Part 2).

Becker, H. (1963) *Outsiders*. New York: Macmillan.

Blot, W. and Tarone, R. (2015) Doll and Peto's quantitative estimates of cancer risks: holding generally true for 35 years. *Journal of the National Cancer Institute*, 107(4): doi.org/10.1093/jnci/djv044.

Bowlby, J. (1953) *Child Care and the Growth of Love*. London: Pelican.

Care Quality Commission (2011) *Care Quality Commission Looks Ahead as Last Count Me In Census is Published*. Available at: www.cqc.org.uk/content/care-quality-commission-looks-ahead-last-count-me-census-published (accessed 10 April 2017).

Cooley, C.H. (1902 [1930]) *Human Nature and the Social Order*. New York: Scribner.

Corr, C., Doka, K. and Kastenbaum, R. (2007) Dying and its interpreters: a review of selected literature and some comments on the state of the field. *Omega: The Journal of Death and Dying*, 39: 239–59.

Cullen, A. (1974) Labelling theory and social deviance. *Journal Perspectives in Psychiatric Care*, 1744–6163.1974.tb01112

Cumming, E. and Earl Henry, W. (1961) *Growing Old*. New York: Basic Books.

Doll, R. and Peto, R. (1981) The causes of cancer: quantitative estimates of risks of cancer in the United States today. *Journal of the National Cancer Institute*, 66(6): 1191–308.

Durkheim, E. (1897 [1951]) *Suicide: A Study in Sociology*. New York: The Free Press.

Engel, G. (1977) The need for a new medical model: a challenge for biomedicine. *Science*, 196(4286): 129–36.

Erikson, E. (1959 [1994]) *Identity and the Life Cycle*. New York: Norton.

Farmer, P. (1999) *Infections and Inequalities: The Modern Plagues*. Berkeley, CA: University of California Press.

Fraley, R. and Shaver, P. (2000) Adult romantic attachment: theoretical developments, emerging controversies, and unanswered questions. *Review of General Psychology*, 4: 132–54.

Freud, S. (2010 [1923]) *The Ego and the Id*. Seattle, WA: Pacific Publishing Studio.

Friedan, B. (1963) *The Feminine Mystique*. London: Victor Gollancz.

Goffman, E. (1963) *Stigma*. London: Penguin.

Havighurst, R. (1963) *Adjustment to Retirement: A Cross-national Study*. Assen, The Netherlands: Van Gorcum.

hooks, b. (2001) Black women: shaping feminist theory. In K. Bhavnani (ed.), *Feminism and 'Race'*. Oxford: Oxford University Press. pp. 33–9.

Hothersall, D. (2003) *History of Psychology*. New York: McGraw–Hill.

Illich, I. (1976) *Limits to Medicine: Medical Nemesis – The Expropriation of Health*. London: Boyers Publishing.

Kastenbaum, R. and Costa, P. (1977) Psychological perspectives on death. *Annual Review of Psychology*, 28: 225–49.

Kenrick, D., Griskevicius V., Neuberg, S. and Schaller, M. (2010) Renovating the pyramid of needs: contemporary extensions built upon ancient foundations. *Perspectives on Psychological Science*, 5(3): 292–314.

Kübler-Ross, E. (1969) *On Death and Dying*. New York: Simon and Schuster.

Kuhn, T. (1962) *The Structure of Scientific Revolutions*. Chicago, IL: University of Chicago Press.

Levinson, D. (1986) *The Seasons of a Man's Life: The Groundbreaking 10-Year Study That Was the Basis for Passages*. London: Random House.

Maslow, A. (1943) Theory of human motivation. *Psychological Review*, 50(4): 370–96.

Mead, G.H. (1934) *Mind, Self and Society: From the Standpoint of a Social Behaviorist* (ed. C.W. Morris). Chicago: University of Chicago Press.

Millett, K. (2000) *Sexual Politics*. Urbana, IL: University of Illinois Press.

Neher, A. (1991) Maslow's theory of motivation: a critique. *Journal of Humanistic Psychology*, 31(3).

Neugarten, B. (1974) Time, age, and the life cycle. *American Journal of Psychiatry*, 136: 887–93.

Parsons, T. (1951) *The Social System*. New York: The Free Press.

Piaget, J. (1953) *Logic and Psychology*. Manchester: Manchester University Press.

Rege, S. (2003) *Sociology of Gender: The Challenge of Feminist Sociological Knowledge*. Thousand Oaks, CA: Sage.

Rogers, C. (1961) *On Becoming a Person*. London: Constable and Robinson.

Schaffer, H.R. (1996) *Social Development*. London: Wiley.

Stacey, M. (1994) The power of lay knowledge: A personal view. In Popay, J. and Williams, G. (eds) *Researching the People's Health*. London: Routledge.

Vaillant, G. (2002) *Aging Well: Surprising Guideposts to a Happier Life from the Landmark Study of Adult Development*. Cambridge, MA: Harvard University Press.

Watson, J. and Rayner, R. (1920) Conditioned emotional reaction. *Journal of Experimental Psychology*, 3: 1–14.

Yeung, K. and Martin, J. (2003) The Looking Glass Self: an empirical test and elaboration. *Social Forces*, 81(3): 843–79.

9

HEALTH PROMOTION

Scott Ellis

To define 'health promotion', students and researchers typically refer to the World Health Organization's (WHO) constitutional definition that health is about a holistic approach to living and not just the prevention of disease. This definition dates back to WHO's inception in 1948 and reflected a bold definition of health for everyone. It is still relevant today of course, but we need a much more responsive and adaptable understanding of health promotion to meet the changing demands on our lives and on our health. People are more mobile than ever before, which brings new challenges in how we address problems such as alcoholism, substance misuse and poor sexual health. This is further exacerbated by the political and economic climates of the Western world, which typically foster elitism and material gain, and vilify the poor and financially vulnerable. This translates into poorer health overall, particularly in relation to obesity, which affects people who live in deprived areas and have lower incomes more frequently than those with a steady income (Public Health England, 2016).

 Glossary

Definitions are provided by the WHO, 2016:

- **Community action for health** The collective efforts by communities which are directed towards increasing community control over the determinants of health, and thereby improving health
- **Disease prevention** Disease prevention covers measures not only to prevent the occurrence of disease, such as risk factor reduction, but also to arrest its progress and reduce its consequences once established
- **Health** As determined by Ottawa Charter for Health Promotion (WHO, 1948)
- **Health education** Concerned with the communication of information, and fostering the motivation, skills and confidence (self-efficacy) necessary to take action to improve health

- **Health promotion** Health promotion is the process of enabling people to increase control over, and to improve their health
- **Health for all** The attainment by all the people of the world of a level of health that will permit them to lead a socially and economically productive life
- **Public health** The science and art of promoting health, preventing disease and prolonging life through the organised efforts of society

INTRODUCTION

In this chapter we will consider the health outcomes for diverse groups of people who are targeted with health promotion campaigns and discuss the efficacy of our most common methods of health promotion. We will also consider health promotion theory and models of practice by examining health promotion campaigns in the UK and in the USA. In addition, we will also consider the effectiveness of shock tactics in health promotion and then consider workplace health promotion in healthcare settings. This chapter asks you to engage in reflective activities as part of your learning journey.

BEHAVIOUR MODIFICATION AND HARM REDUCTION

Behaviour modification and harm reduction are the most common aims of health promotion (see Figure 9.1), through improving policy, mobilising community action and using social marketing techniques to communicate with a defined target audience (Glasgow et al., 2004; Michie and Abraham, 2004; Whitehead, 2004). Mass media is a simple social marketing technique that can be used to expose large numbers of people to a targeted message and image. This often takes the form of posters, magazine and newspaper advertising and television and radio adverts. Small media uses similar techniques such as print booklets or pocket-sized information cards. Digital media has become increasingly common as a method to reach and engage with a target audience, particularly in sexual health work with young people, who value privacy and efficient access to advice (Bailey et al., 2015).

In all of these methods, there are elements that can be tailored to reach individuals within a population group given some extra planning and scoping of an area. The campaign shown in Figure 9.2 was part of a health promotion campaign to empower women to take control of their sexual health as an HIV prevention and education strategy in the USA. The focal point of the campaign is a confident Black woman and large posters such as this were displayed in neighbourhoods across New York City where HIV incidence rates were high and where census information showed there to be a high proportion of Black female residents.

While advertising can be placed in the press based on a magazine or newspaper's known readership, this is far from an exact art. For instance, most of the UK's press aimed at gay men is saturated by HIV prevention work, which makes it difficult for

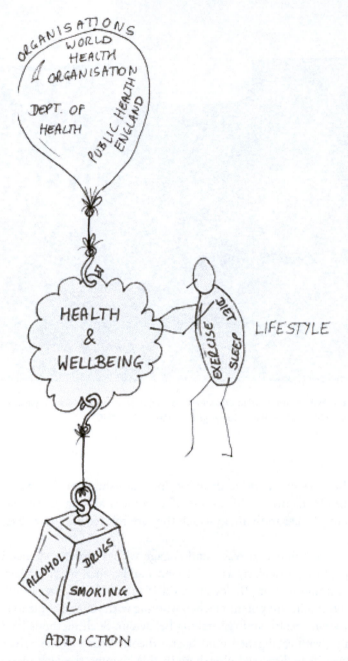

Figure 9.1   Health and wellbeing

health promoters to know how many people read or understand their work. Similarly, health promotion advertising in bars and clubs is common, including NHS-driven safer drinking campaigns. Such approaches seek to meet WHO's healthy settings approach to health promotion (2016), but do not address the disparity between

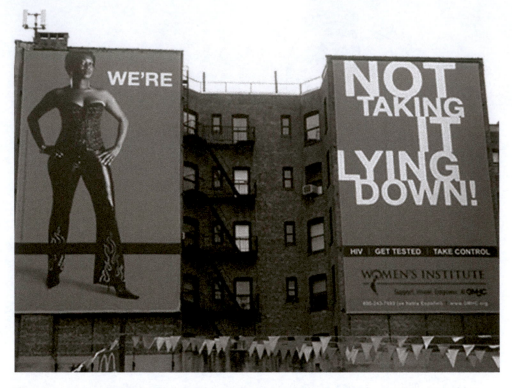

Figure 9.2   *We're Not Taking It Lying Down!* HIV prevention campaign for Gay Men's Health Crisis, Women's Institute at GMHC. Copyright courtesy of GMHC

advertising the risks of excessive drinking in establishments that exist to promote this. Dooris (2009) identifies this as less of a problem as long as we reach people in an environment familiar to them, in which they are relaxed and more likely to engage with stimuli.

Using digital techniques to reach and engage with a target audience is becoming increasingly popular, particularly as social media and e-mail provide platforms rich in user behavioural information. Bailey et al. (2015) identified digital health promotion methods to have significant potential when working with young people to improve their knowledge of sexual health and risk-taking behaviour. Such methods lend themselves well to planning with established models and theories, such as the behaviour-change theory. However, as is discussed elsewhere in this chapter, the lack of current multi-agency, cross-sector working in the UK's health sector hinders our ability to fully utilise the possibilities of digital health promotion at present. Despite this, some health promotion organisations and NHS centres use digital methods for engagement, including to communicate sexual health screening results and to enable young people to access sexual health advice and condoms.

Key challenges

Which health problems to prioritise for intervention, and which population groups to target, are often dictated by national epidemiological data. In the UK, the Office for National Statistics monitors morbidity and mortality data that show us where problems with disease incidence lie and who is affected most prominently by avoidable poor health outcomes. Most commonly, this relates to health inequalities such as poor access to healthcare for people with lower levels of education, or those who live in poverty and with unemployment. However, a key challenge for all of those who work in health promotion is how to balance this sensibly with the needs of people who do not live in poverty or in areas of deprivation. This can often be a challenging concept for students to comprehend as the news media and social marketing frequently present minority groups as the most in need.

Indeed, we know that wealth or income are linked on a gradient with health. For instance, as income levels rise, significant health risks decline (Woolf et al., 2015). Similarly, the more income a person has, the more likely they are to describe their own health as good (Schiller et al., 2012). However, some health problems and risks transcend levels of wealth or poverty and by focusing health promotion only on groups most visibly in need, we risk missing an opportunity to engage with people who are in need of urgent intervention. A key example is suicide risk amongst men, regardless of their social background or financial standing.

Suicide is the seventh leading cause of death for men in Canada (Bilsker and White, 2011) and the USA (CDC, 2015), and the twelfth leading cause of death in the UK (ONS, 2015). Societal pressures placed on men that dictate norms of constructed masculinity, including an aversion to showing emotion or demonstrating empathy, contribute significantly to these data (Bilsker and White, 2011). There have been recent drives to address the unmet needs of men in general, and young White men specifically in both the USA and the UK. For instance the Write Home Project was set up as a non-profit organisation to help homeless youth in the Berkeley, California, area by utilising art and clinic spaces to provide holistic activities that support wellbeing. The project's polished, emotionally charged resources have provided effective discussion points for health promotion students in exploring how to move beyond simplistic mass media posters when addressing the most vulnerable in society.

With similarities to the ethos of honesty and transparent communication promoted by the *Write Home Project*, Mark Henick, a speaker at TedX Toronto in 2013, spoke candidly about his experience of a suicide attempt. He very clearly describes the events leading up to his attempt to end his own life and forges a clear pathway for health promoters in how to prevent those under their care from the same risks. Both examples demonstrate how we can better engage with people at all social, economic and political levels of society whilst avoiding the narrow-mindedness that often occurs naturally when relying excessively on data from a single source or from biased organisations.

Theories and models

Raingruber (2014) cites a number of health researchers who identify significant gaps in the conceptual framework or theoretical basis of health promotion campaigns. This most commonly happens when individual agencies have a lack of researcher expertise or have a remit to fulfil a narrow agenda. Raingruber identifies 18 distinct health promotion theories and models based on various areas of research and development and that can be chosen for individual campaigns based on the planned goals and outcomes. Criticism of the use of theories and models does exist, but is commonly centred on the failure of health promoters to fully utilise the potential of theoretical constructs (Eccles et al., 2005) or to implement the model components (Merzel and D'Afflitti, 2003) rather than failures of the models themselves.

Models range from the simplistic, such as the health belief model (HBM) with its six constructs, to the complex, such as the precede–proceed model (PPM), which has ten constructs within an eight-phase process. I have found few constants in how the hundreds of students I have supervised have chosen their preferred health model or theory, other than they work from the basis of whether they intrinsically believe in a particular medical or social approach to health improvement. A variety of researchers deconstruct this further, and believe the choice of model or theory is less important than the need to integrate multiple constructs in health promotion (Best et al., 2003), as identified by Suls and Rothman (2004) in the biopsychosocial model. (You can read more about the biopsychosocial model in Chapter 8, Applied Health Sciences.) McGinnis et al. (2002) based the likely success or failure of a health promotion campaign on its leadership, which cannot perform meaningfully or efficiently if the work is not grounded in a theoretical and conceptual framework.

The Stages of Community Readiness model is adaptable to multiple health promotion contexts and which students have found accessible (Figure 9.3). Most useful in the early stages of campaign planning, the model has similarities to Corcoran's (2007) nine stages planning model and includes scope for the on-going development of a campaign into professional fields or long-term responsive placement. The Stages of Community Readiness model is used as part of a 'Community Tool Box' developed by the Work Group for Community Health and Development at the University of Kansas (2015) and can be used to position a health promotion campaign within specific communities based on their existing knowledge of a health problem or threat.

Aside from the established academic models and theories readily available for health promoters, professional and non-profit organisations often construct their own framework based on their specialist work. Similarly, individual research projects of all sizes often result in new theories or models ready for further testing.

Figure 9.4 shows the HIV epidemiological triangle, a visually evolved representation of Royce et al.'s (1997) research of contributing factors to HIV transmission. The UK's Terrence Higgins Trust (THT), a non-profit organisation, and the US Centre for Disease Control and Prevention have adopted this model. The model assists

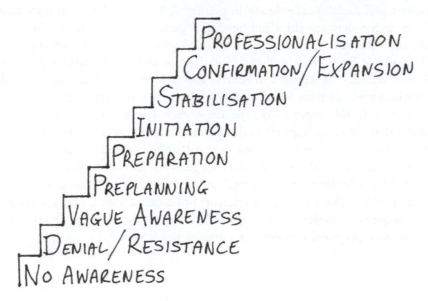

Figure 9.3 Stages of Community Readiness model, University of Kansas

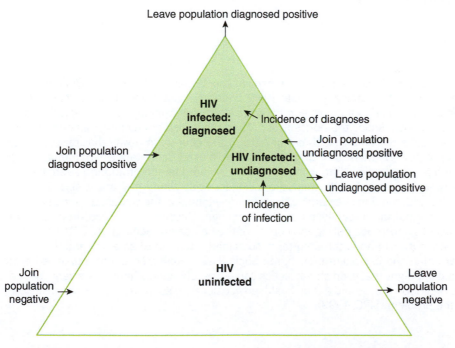

Figure 9.4 HIV among MSM in England. HIV epidemiological triangle, THT. Copyright: Ford Hickson makingitcount.org 2016

researchers and health professionals in predicting HIV incidence rates by analysing local population demographics and behaviour patterns. Similar to the Stages of the Community Readiness model, the epidemiological triangle is particularly useful to scholars as it lends itself well to adaptations to address different areas of health. Addiction, sexually transmitted infections and domestic violence are all conditions that previous students have found useful to frame using this representation.

Fried et al. (2004) reported on the Experience Corps programme in Baltimore, Maryland that aimed to improve health promotion amongst an ageing population by using a social approach to reduce risk factors that are known to cause disability and other preventable morbidities. The paper suggests the use of the Experience Corps as a social model of health promotion, application of which can be useful in supporting a population with multiple health risks that are often unaddressed. This is a good example of how active, community-based research can generate novel approaches to health promotion to supplement contemporary approaches.

Go Further 9.1

You can read more about this initiative at:

www.aarp.org/experience-corps/experience-corps-volunteer/experience-corps-cities-baltimore.html

Case Study 9.1

The Thatcher Conservative government of the 1980s released the now infamous *Don't Die of Ignorance* campaign in late 1986. Widely criticised since then for its demonisation of sex, particularly amongst non-heterosexuals, the campaign was nevertheless instrumental in introducing the concept of AIDS to the British population. Although this served to introduce the emerging threat of AIDS to the country in a way that made it clear this was not just an American – or gay – problem, it used 'scare tactics' to dramatise a public health problem rather than using structured, tailored health promotion strategies to raise awareness. Sexual health counsellors working with young gay and bisexual people are familiar with the damage caused to sexual development and welfare as a result of the fear and marginalisation catalysed by the campaign. Despite a recorded drop in diagnosed cases of gonorrhoea during the course of the campaign (Seña et al., 2010), there is little evidence it resulted in the long-term, sustained adoption of safe sex practices. Thirteen years after the campaign launch, the Social Issues Research Centre published evidence that campaigns that used shock tactics caused psychological harm to viewers and reduced the likelihood they would act on health advice because such campaigns desensitised them to the problem (SIRC, 1999).

More recent research maintains health promotion that uses social marketing as a delivery channel typically fails to address longstanding ethical concerns with such tactics, including whether the intended outcome can be justified through means designed to induce fear (Slavin et al., 2007). Activists and social workers have also been vocal about the lack of evidence of measurable impact or efficacy from intentionally scaring people. Bill Ryan, a health activist, psychotherapist and professor of social work, identifies the 'packaging' – or the imagery and language – of such campaigns as particularly problematic for young people, as it simply represents a recycling of concepts that have tenuous links to successful harm reduction (CATIE, 2011). Measurement of behaviour change as a result of health promotion campaigns varies from 3% to 17% depending on the source and type (Snyder and Hamilton, 2002; Snyder et al., 2004) and is rarely attributed to shock tactics.

Go Further 9.2

You can find the SIRC report at www.sirc.org/news/sideeffects.html.

DO SHOCK TACTICS WORK?

Although the positioning of shock tactics within health promotion and social marketing strategies remains unresolved, the health sector's failure to address sexually transmitted HIV and the emergence of related high-risk behaviours translates to repeated experimentation with controversial, eye-catching imagery.

In response to the increasing incidence of sexually transmitted HIV amongst men who have sex with men (MSM) in Canada in 2004, AIDS Vancouver, alongside a number of national health agencies and authorities, released the *Think Again* campaign (Figure 9.5). The campaign designers used sexually graphic, eye-catching imagery to draw attention to the fact HIV is often transmitted because sexual partners are unaware of the other's status. The campaign was based on established knowledge of how men negotiated sexual risk, as well as the outcomes of focus groups facilitated by an expert in the field. Interestingly, they did not use a recognised health promotion model in its design (Lombardo and Léger, 2007). Although some religious and other community groups criticised the sexually graphic imagery, which they equated to shock tactics, the visual representation of the psychosocial principles of sexual activity (Maibach et al., 1993) developed the more common social marketing approach of delivering a message that communicates an ultimate 'endpoint'.

An outcome assessment exercise of the *Think Again* campaign showed promise with the innovative use of explicit graphics without a direct or intentional shock value. The evaluation took into account the views of 417 men to whom the campaign was targeted. In this sample, 73% of men said they found the campaign 'appealing' and 76% said they reconsidered their sexual practices as a result. In addition, 48% said they had changed 'something' about their sexual practices as a result, with men reporting high-risk sexual behaviour more likely to reconsider their behaviour. This suggests renewed health

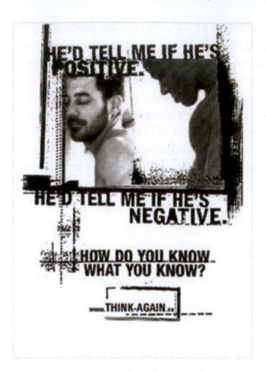

Figure 9.5   Sample poster from the *Think Again* campaign. Copyright Dr Brian Chittock, AIDS Vancouver

promotion efforts to address well-established, longitudinal health problems may well be effective if their use of explicit imagery and messages is socioculturally appropriate, regardless of the potential cause for offence in other social groups.

Health promotion researchers, academics, students and practitioners have no shortage of material from which to assess the efficacy of such campaigns. There is little, however, to suggest we can approach all controversial or 'shocking' material from the same point of view. While the judgement that some imagery is inherently distasteful or offensive (Guttman and Salmon, 2004) may well be valid, evaluations of individual campaigns force us to consider potential and impact on a case-by-case basis, as is shown by *Think Again*. By their very nature, campaigns that force us to consider our sexual behaviour often use explicit imagery and language to get a point across, thus inviting criticism on the grounds of taste and social acceptability. Smoking cessation, mental health and drink driving campaigns have all tried to shock or scare people to engage them and instigate meaningful behaviour change.

In 2005, the Thomas and Stacey Siebel Foundation and the Partnership for Drug-Free Kids launched *The Meth Project* in Montana, USA in response to US Department of Justice data that methamphetamine ('meth') use amongst young people was increasing. The project describes its campaign imagery as 'hard-hitting' and typically shows either a teenager at the point of deciding whether to try meth for the first time or in

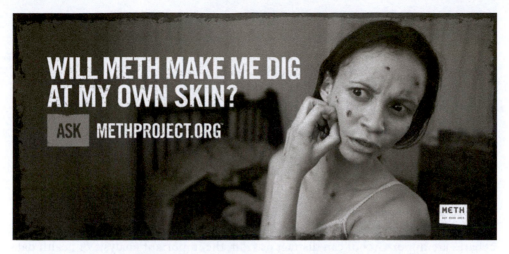

Figure 9.6   Campaign poster from The Meth Project (methproject.org, 2016). Copyright Teri Christensen at drugfree.org

a situation related to their addiction. Scenarios include a boy violently robbing his parents' house with two friends, a teenage girl having sex with a man in a motel, supervised by her boyfriend, and a teenage boy offering a much older man oral sex. All three scenarios centre on the main character trying to steal or earn money to be able to buy meth along with a strapline that tells us that doing so is normal when you are addicted to meth. Figure 9.6 is an example of one of the many engaging, if controversial, images of the project.

The Meth Project has partnered with state health authorities and as of 2016 is active in six states and has evaluated the efficacy and impact of the project through surveys involving over 50,000 teenagers and 112 focus groups (Meth Project Foundation, 2016). Several statutory organisations recorded significant changes in meth use and health outcomes since the project launched. This includes a significant change in Montana's national ranking for meth use from number five in the country in 2005 to 39 in 2011 (Office of National Drug Control Policy) and a 65% reduction in meth use amongst teenagers in Arizona was reported by the Arizona Criminal Justice Commission in the four years after the project was launched there in 2006 (Arizona Criminal Justice Commission, 2010).

Go Further 9.3

You can research The Meth Project at www.methproject.org

Lecturers have used these digital resources in health promotion campaigns with undergraduate and postgraduate discussion groups amongst health promotion and public health students with varying outcomes. Most students agreed the imagery was eye-catching and caught their attention, and many students thought it was an appropriate response to a recreational drug that is highly addictive. Between 2005 and 2011, the project also won 41 media awards and the Stanford Graduate School of Business Center praised the campaign for its philanthropic approach to addressing an urgent social problem. Unlike Ryan's (CATIE, 2011) concern that shocking consumers of health messages creates a barrier between the individual and the core message, Morales et al. (2012) found the 'disgust' factor in the Meth Project's campaign, such as rotting teeth and infected skin sores, resulted in teenagers establishing a distance between themselves and the behaviour associated with the disgusting images, in this case the use of meth.

Much attention is paid to the design, imagery and content of mass media health promotion campaigns, and there is ample scope for debates on the appropriateness of pictures designed to provoke a response or catalyse a behaviour change. Such debates are important but can distract us from the important analysis of health data that enables us to more accurately assess the need for a campaign and its effects. Anderson (2010) demonstrates this with an analysis of national meth use data using the Youth Risk Behaviour Surveys and concludes that the Meth Project had no discernible impact on meth use. Indeed, the research finds meth use was declining at the start of the project and simply maintained this trajectory. The multiple awards given to the campaign as well as its state-level recognition and substantial funding warn us of the risk and to consider both the reception a campaign gets, as well as its demonstrable effects.

⚙️ Activity 9.1

The private, statutory and non-profit sectors are unlikely partners in health promotion. The disparities between generating a profit, establishing and achieving commissioning targets, and making a difference in a community represent so many competing priorities and goals, that it is surprising multi-sector campaigns ever get off the ground. In 2008, I joined the multi-agency *Pan-London HIV Prevention Programme* (PLHPP). The UK's Department for Health commissioned the programme to address rising HIV incidence amongst MSM and Black Africans. As the lead for gay men's mass media, I found myself negotiating media design and messages between the very disparate partners involved. The first concern was that the project mandate assumed that Black Africans and MSM were mutually exclusive. This made it difficult to justify to budget-holders why mass media should be fully representative of London's very diverse populations. For example, if we showed two Black men kissing in a poster, should the billing and evaluation be attributed to the Black African part of the project or the MSM part of the project? A definitive answer was not forthcoming. A private sector firm, with no experience in sexual health, evaluated the project. They heavily criticised the data we could provide based on market saturation of mass media market. Although we knew how many press adverts we had placed, and what the monthly distribution of the magazines were, we did not know how many people picked up a magazine, saw our adverts, paid attention to them or understood them.

Why do you think it was difficult for a non-profit and a private sector organisation to work together on this project? Write some notes before reading the discussion.

AUTOETHNOGRAPHIC EXPERIENCES IN HEALTH PROMOTION

How then, are we to navigate the complex political, economic and social structures that influence health promotion work so closely? Multi-agency working is not something historically equated with statutory agencies and authorities in the UK. Some agencies have begun to recognise the need for more efficient collaborative work in health since the end of the PLHPP in 2011. In 2014, the National Institute of Health and Care Excellence (NICE) released a guidance document for multi-agency working with people who experience domestic violence and abuse. Also in 2014, the Home Office released guidance on multi-agency working and information sharing for agencies involved in safeguarding. Both documents highlight the need for transparent communication and a shared model of work and practice. We did not have a shared model of work during the PLHPP, but instead spent a great deal of time locked in discussions about how to interpret behavioural data on the sexual patterns of MSM and Black Africans. This highlighted differences of opinion and professional judgement in how to reach our target groups. We knew that community leaders and church leaders were key to reaching Black Africans, and the gay press, bars and clubs were important in reaching MSM. We also based our work on established research and models. Engel's (1977) biopsychosocial model was key to our design and implementation strategy. Merzel and D'Afflitti (2003) asserted that the most effective campaigns are community-based, where they target large groups for intervention. This study also highlighted HIV prevention as the most likely to succeed in behaviour change, compared with health promotion based on cardiovascular disease, cancer, smoking cessation and substance use.

Combining our evidence base with a strategy to engage people involved with African community centres, the managers of gay bars and the editors of magazines was central to a plan to ensure the PLHPP was advertised as broadly as possible. Anecdotally, this was received more positively in African community centres and churches than it was in gay bars and clubs. This seemed to be because it was a novel topic in an African community environment not normally associated with sexual health discussions. However, gay bars are typically saturated with sexualised media and competing messages from numerous health promotion agencies and authorities. As such, our messages were somewhat diluted by the environment and it was not clear if they had an impact. As one of the non-profit agencies involved in the PLHPP, we used the gravitas of our brand name to demonstrate to readers within our target group that we were working with the NHS and not with for-profit healthcare services. Participants in focus groups we held to gauge response to the campaign design raised these as important factors, and said they would be more willing to trust the message if our branding was used in conjunction with the NHS logo. Working in the PLHPP highlighted the need for more collaboration amongst the various agencies in HIV prevention as well as the need for a more robust model in which private and non-profit sector agencies can work together meaningfully to stimulate behaviour change.

HEALTH PROMOTION IN HEALTHCARE SETTINGS

In an effort to establish benchmarks for safe practice and effective patient outcomes, the Care Quality Commission is mandated nationally to inspect all healthcare services using a regulatory and compliance model. This encourages providers of health services to ensure their practice is person-centred and provided in the safest manner possible. It penalises poor performance and rewards the best providers by enabling them to promote their services on the basis of their proven track record. This model provides an interesting context within which to consider how health promotion can be embedded in primary and secondary healthcare services, rather than relying predominantly on community-based interventions led by non-profit agencies. With increasing national recognition that individuals are attending hospitals, and their family doctors in reaction to preventable conditions that result from behaviours such as excessive alcohol consumption and obesity, greater focus has been placed on frontline health professionals to engage patients with health promotion messages (Bennett et al., 2009; Simon, 2012).

Healthcare staff and health promotion

The Royal College of Nursing (RCN) recognised the opportunity for their members to become more involved in public health and, in 2012, published a policy document aimed at reducing the reliance on the NHS as a 'sickness service' (Royal College of Nursing, 2012: 3). In setting out evidence-based recommendations for national practice, the RCN utilised case studies from nurses in all four UK countries to demonstrate the impact clinical staff can have on health outcomes in areas more commonly associated with health promotion, such as breast and cervical screening and sexual health. In doing so the organisation has identified how vulnerable or high-risk groups can be reached through a variety of clinical and community settings that extend the basic premise of mass media health promotion. Health professionals' experiences in regulation have shown many innovative examples of how frontline health staff have tried to combine immediate treatment with longer-term health promotion. This includes decorating a hospital inpatient ward in a dementia-friendly style to show relatives how they could adapt their home to make it a safer space, and an emergency department that employed a team of social workers within the department 24 hours a day to meet the needs of a teenage population with escalating substance misuse.

 Activity 9.2

Reflect on your working environment. How can a health promotion message be integrated into your working day? Relate this to Chapter 4, Leadership and Teamwork. Can you take a leadership role on promoting health?

A series of child deaths as a result of the failure of different authorities and agencies to work together led to serious case reviews of practice, all of which identified how more collaborative, transparent working could have prevented the deaths of abused children. In a similar way, health promoters must accept that mass media campaigns continually recycled by non-profit agencies could benefit from a multidisciplinary approach that involves the professionals in the sector responsible for treating the health problems the campaign work seeks to prevent in the first place.

CHAPTER SUMMARY

- As we live in ever-more diversified communities, so we begin to understand how global movement, behaviour change and sociopolitical conditions affect how we view our health and that of our community.
- Simple, proven models of health promotion based on perception of risk and rewards for behaviour change do not easily meet the increasingly complex needs of people with multiple health risks or those who accept risky choices as a typical part of their lifestyle.
- Although existing research frameworks for health interventions rarely indicate that scare or shock tactics are successful in facilitating improved outcomes, health promoters and social marketers are often drawn to recycle such approaches in an anxious attempt to address urgent health problems.
- Adaptations of such tactics that include explicit text and images, often around sexual activity, drug use or behaviour likely to cause significant harm to others, are often arguably more successful than approaches that simply induce fear.
- This may be because visually explicit campaigns attract attention without inherently repelling people with threats. Instead, the reader recognises their own behaviour or lifestyle in the imagery presented, particularly if it delivers a non-judgemental and uncontrived message.
- In such circumstances, individuals can reflect and consider their risks at their own pace and in the context of the activities and choices that are important to them. In this sense, health promoters should prioritise work that catalyses a thinking reaction from those whose behaviour or risks concern them most.

📖 FURTHER READING

Websites

- The World Health Organization: www.who.int
- Public Health England: www.gov.uk/government/organisations/public-health-england
- Royal College of Nursing: www.rcn.org.uk
- NHS: www.nhs.uk

Texts

- Addiction.com (2015) *Celebrating 10 Years of 'Unselling' Meth* [image online]. Available at: www.addiction.com/8061/montana-meth-project-10-year-anniversary/ (accessed 10 August 2016).
- Bailey, J., Mann, S., Wayal, S., Hunter, R., Free, C. and Abraham, C. (2015) Sexual health promotion for young people delivered via digital media: a scoping review. *Public Health Research*, 3(13).
- Bennett, C., Perry, J. and Lawrence, Z. (2009) Health promotion in primary care *Nursing Standard*, 23(47): 48–56.
- Dooris, M. (2009) Holistic and sustainable health improvement: the contribution of the settings-based approach to health promotion. *Perspectives in Public Health*, 129: 29–36.
- Home Office (2014) *Multi Agency Working and Information Sharing Project*. Available at: www.gov.uk/government/uploads/system/uploads/attachment_data/file/338875/MASH.pdf (accessed 25 August 2016).
- Kemppainen, V., Tossavainen, K. and Turunen, H. (2012) Nurses' roles in health promotion practice: an integrative review. *Health Promotion International*, 28(4): 490–501.
- Raingruber, B. (2014) Health promotion theories. In *Contemporary Health Promotion in Nursing Practice*. Burlington, MA: Jones & Bartlett Learning.
- Royal College of Nursing (2012) *Going Upstream: Nursing's Contribution to Public Health*. Available at: www2.rcn.org.uk/__data/assets/pdf_file/0007/433699/004203.pdf (accessed 10 August 2016).
- Slavin, S., Batrouney, C. and Murphy, D. (2007) Fear appeals and treatment side-effects: An effective combination for HIV prevention? *AIDS Care*, 19(1): 130–7.
- The Meth Project (2011) *Project Overview*. Available from http://foundation.methproject.org/documents/Meth%20Project%20Fact%20Sheet%2012-15-11.pdf (accessed 1 August 2016).
- Work Group for Community Health and Development, University of Kansas (2015) *Conducting Concerns Surveys*. Community Tool Box. Available at: http://ctb.ku.edu/en/table-of-contents/assessment/assessing-community-needs-and-resources/conduct-concerns-surveys/main.%C2%A0 (accessed 10 August 2016).

- Witte, K. and Allen, M. (2000) A meta-analysis of fear appeals: implications for effective public health campaigns. *Health Education and Behavior*, 27(5): 591–615.
- World Health Organization (2016) *Introduction to Healthy Settings.* Available at: www.who.int/healthy_settings/about/en/ (accessed 25 August 2016).

REFERENCES

Anderson, D.M. (2010) Does information matter? The effect of the Meth Project on meth use among youths. *Journal of Health Economics*, 29(5): 732–42.

Bailey, J., Mann, S., Wayal, S., Hunter, R., Free, C. and Abraham, C. (2015) Sexual health promotion for young people delivered via digital media: a scoping review. *Public Health Research*, 3(13).

Bennett, C., Perry, J. and Lawrence, Z. (2009) Health promotion in primary care. *Nursing Standard*, 23(47): 48–56.

Best, A., Stokols, D., Green, L., Leischow, S., Holmes, B. and Buchholz, K. (2003) An integrative framework for community partnering to translate theory into effective health promotion strategy. *American Journal of Health Promotion*, 18(2): 168–76.

Bilsker, D. and White, J. (2011) The silent epidemic of male suicide. *British Columbia Medical Journal*, 53(10): 529–34.

CATIE (2011) *Prevention in Focus: Spotlight on Programming and Research* [online]. Available at: www.catie.ca/en/pif/fall-2011/views-front-lines-fear-based-campaigns (accessed 16 August 2016).

CDC (Centers for Disease Control and Prevention) (2015) *Leading Causes of Death in Males United States 2013* [online]. Available at: www.cdc.gov/men/lcod/2013/index.htm (accessed 17 August 2016).

Corcoran, N. (ed.) (2007) *Communicating Health: Strategies for Health Promotion.* London: Sage.

Dooris, M. (2009) Holistic and sustainable health improvement: the contribution of the settings-based approach to health promotion. *Perspectives in Public Health*, 129: 29–36.

Eccles, M., Grimshaw, J., Walker, A., Johnstond, M. and Pittse, N. (2005) Changing the behavior of healthcare professionals: the use of theory in promoting the uptake of research findings. *Journal of Clinical Epidemiology*, 58: 107–112.

Engel, G. (1977) The need for a new medical model: a challenge for biomedicine. *Science*, 196: 129–36.

Fried, L.P., Carlson, M.C., Freedman, M., Frick, K.D., Glass, T.A., Hill, J., McGill, S., Rebok, G.W., Seeman, T., Tielsch, J., Wasik, B.A. and Zeger, S. (2004) A social model for health promotion for an aging population: initial evidence on the experience corps model. *Journal of Urban Health*, 81(1): 64–78.

Glasgow, R.E., Goldstein, M.G., Ockene, J. and Pronk, N.P. (2004) Translating what we have learned into practice: principles and hypotheses for addressing multiple behaviors in primary care. *American Journal of Preventive Medicine*, 27: 88–101.

Guttman, N. and Salmon, C.T. (2004) Guilt, fear, stigma and knowledge gaps: ethical issues in public health communication interventions. *Bioethics*, 18(6): 531–52.

Home Office (2014) *Multi Agency Working and Information Sharing Project.* Available at: www.gov.uk/government/uploads/system/uploads/attachment_data/file/338875/MASH.pdf (accessed 25 August 2017).

Lombardo, A.P. and Léger, Y.A. (2007) Thinking about 'Think Again' in Canada: assessing a social marketing HIV/AIDS prevention campaign *Journal of Health Communication*, 22(4): 377–97.

Maibach, E.W., Kreps, G. and Bonaguro, E.W. (1993). Developing strategic communication campaigns for HIV–AIDS prevention. In S. C. Ratzan (ed.), *AIDS: Effective Health Communication for the 90s*. Washington, DC: Taylor & Francis. pp. 15–35.

McGinnis, J.M., Williams-Russo, P. and Knickman, J.R. (2002) The case for more active policy attention to health promotion. *Health Affairs*, 21(2): 78–93.

Merzel, C. and D'Afflitti, J. (2003) Reconsidering community-based health promotion: promise, performance, and potential. *American Journal of Public Health*, 93(4): 557–74.

Michie, S. and Abraham, C. (2004) Interventions to change health behaviours: evidence-based or evidence-inspired? *Psychology & Health*, 19(1): 29–49.

Morales, A.C., Wu, E.C. and Fitzsimons, G.J. (2012) How disgust enhances the effectiveness of fear appeals. *Journal of Marketing Research*, 49(3): 383–93.

National Institute for Health and Care Excellence (2014) Domestic violence and abuse: multi-agency working: guidance (PH50). Available at: www.nice.org.uk/guidance/ph50 (accessed 25 August 2016).

ONS (Office for National Statistics) (2015) What are the top causes of death by age and gender? Available at: http://visual.ons.gov.uk/what-are-the-top-causes-of-death-by-age-and-gender/ (accessed 14 March 2017).

Public Health England (2016) *Health Inequalities*. Available at: www.noo.org.uk/NOO_about_obesity/inequalities (accessed 10 April 2017).

Raingruber, B. (2014) Health promotion theories. In *Contemporary Health Promotion in Nursing Practice*. Burlington, MA: Jones & Bartlett Learning.

Royal College of Nursing (2012) *Going Upstream: Nursing's Contribution to Public Health*. Available at: www2.rcn.org.uk/__data/assets/pdf_file/0007/433699/004203.pdf (accessed 10 August 2016).

Royce, R.A., Seña, A., Cates, W. and Cohen, M.S. (1997) Sexual transmission of HIV. *New England Journal of Medicine*, 337: 799.

Schiller, J.S., Lucas, J.W. and Peregoy, J.A. (2012) *Summary Health Statistics for U.S. Adults: National Health Interview Survey, 2011. Vital and Health Statistics 10 (256): Table 21*. Available at: www.cdc.gov/nchs/data/series/sr_10/sr10_256.pdf (accessed 9 August 2016).

Seña, A.C., Hammer, J.P., Wilson, K., Zeveloff, A. and Gamble, J. (2010) Feasibility and acceptability of door-to-door rapid HIV testing among Latino immigrants and their HIV risk factors in North Carolina. *AIDS Patient Care and STDs*, 24(3): 165–73.

Simon, C. (2012) Health Promotion in primary care. *InnovAiT*, 5(12): 725–31.

Slavin, S., Batrouney, C. and Murphy, D. (2007) Fear appeals and treatment side-effects: An effective combination for HIV prevention? *AIDS Care*, 19(1): 130–7.

SIRC (Social Issues Research Centre) (1999) The side effects of health warnings [online]. Available at: www.sirc.org/news/side.pdf (accessed 9 August 2016).

Snyder, L.B. and Hamilton, M.A. (2002) Meta-analysis of US health campaign effects on behavior, emphasize enforcement, exposure and new information and beware the secular trend. In R. Horrick (ed.), *Public Health Communication: Evidence for Behavior Change*. Hillsdale, NJ: Lawrence Erlbaum. pp. 357–83.

Snyder, L.B. and Hamilton, M.A., Mitchell, E.W. Kiwanuka-Tondo, J., Fleming-Milici, F. and Proctor, D.A. (2004) Meta-analysis of the effect of mediated health communication campaigns on behavior change in the United States. *Journal of Health Communication*, 9(Suppl 1): 71–96.

Suls, J. and Rothman, A. (2004) Evolution of the biopsychosocial model: prospects and challenges for health psychology. *Journal of Health Psychology*, 23(2): 119–25.

The Meth Project Foundation (2016) Project Overview [online]. Available at: http://foundation.methproject.org/documents/Meth%20Project%20Fact%20Sheet%2012-15-11.pdf (accessed 1 August 2016).

Whitehead, D. (2004) Health promotion and health education: advancing the concepts. *Journal of Advanced Nursing*, 47(3): 311–20.

Woolf, S.H., Aron, L., Dubay, L., Simon, S.M., Zimmerman, E. and Luk, K.X. (2015) *How are Income and Wealth Linked to Health and Longevity? Income and Health Initiative: Brief One.* Available at: www.urban.org/sites/default/files/alfresco/publication-pdfs/2000178-How-are-Income-and-Wealth-Linked-to-Health-and-Longevity.pdf (accessed 1 September 2016).

World Health Organization (1948) *Ottawa Charter for Health Promotion.* Geneva: WHO.

World Health Organization (2016) *Introduction to Healthy Settings.* Available at: www.who.int/healthy_settings/about/en/ (accessed 25 August 2016).

Work Group for Community Health and Development, University of Kansas (2015) *Conducting Concerns Surveys. Community Tool Box.* Available at: http://ctb.ku.edu/en/table-of-contents/assessment/assessing-community-needs-and-resources/conduct-concerns-surveys/main.%C2%A0 (accessed 10 August 2016).

Write Home Project (2014) *Broken Bottles* [video online]. Available at: www.youtube.com/watch?v=O2senVu65JQ (accessed 1 August 2016).

PART THREE

WORKING WITH DIFFERENT GROUPS OF PEOPLE

10

ADDITIONAL NEEDS AND CHALLENGING BEHAVIOURS IN ADULTS AND CHILDREN

Kevin Graham

Remember, no-one can make you feel inferior without your consent.

Eleanor Roosevelt

This chapter introduces you to theories that explain additional needs and challenging behaviours. It will consider what these terms mean and how they are used in settings to describe and explain various cognitive disabilities and how such disabilities can result in challenging behaviour. Disabled people suffer from not just their disability but the prejudice that society expresses and this chapter will help you to understand how stereotyping can impact on people's self-esteem. You will also consider legal and ethical frameworks in which your practice takes place.

Glossary

- **Additional needs** A need for additional support
- **ADHD** Attention deficit hyperactivity disorder
- **Behavioural, emotional and social difficulties (BESD) and social, emotional and mental health (SEMH)** Someone with an adjustment disorder such as obsessive–compulsory disorder (OCD) or has disruptive, anti-social and aggressive behaviour
- **Challenging behaviour** Culturally abnormal behaviour
- **Dementia** A cluster of symptoms relating to memory loss

(Continued)

(Continued)

- **Disability** A substantial long-term physical or mental impairment
- **Dyslexia** Difficulty in learning to read or interpret words or other symbols; does not affect general intelligence
- **Learning disability/difficulty** Reduced intellectual ability
- **SEN** Special Educational Needs

INTRODUCTION

As caregivers, we need to gain an understanding of how our responses to additional needs and challenging behaviours are informed by a combination of theoretical and practical models. It is also important for any aspiring practitioner to develop their own understanding of inclusion in workbased settings. This chapter will help you to understand a range of approaches, linked to best practice, and develop your recognition of the causes of challenging behaviours.

Scenario 10.1

David is a 14-year-old boy. Although short and obese, he has a usually friendly nature. He suffers from Prader–Willi syndrome and has autistic tendencies. He is sensitive to noise and picks his skin when anxious. David is assessed as SEN and has a higher level teaching assistant to support him. David is frequently teased as he is cross-eyed, this leads to anger outbursts, which if not mediated quickly, can deteriorate into violence towards his tormenter.

- Can you think how David can be supported and what strategies could be used to prevent his anger outbursts?
- Write down your ideas and then revisit your writing after you have read the chapter.

ADDITIONAL NEEDS

How do we consider a service user to have what we would describe as an 'additional need'? We would start by acknowledging that a service user could be identified as falling within what is termed 'atypical development'. This means development does not follow the recognised pattern seen in most people and therefore would result in the individual needing some form of support to ensure they are able to access the same opportunities as everyone else.

Please note: The term *additional needs* is often used interchangeably with the commonly used *special needs*, which would mean an individual or service user ordinarily requires support to enable them to partake in day-to-day activities.

The use of the term Special Educational Needs (SEN) denotes that a learner has a greater difficulty in learning than most children of his/her age:

A Child has SEN if they have a learning difficulty which calls for special educational provision to be made for them. (Education Act 1996; Special Educational Needs and Disability Act [SENDA] 2001)

Provision to support someone with SEN is generally defined relative to the provision that is normally available. However, for adult service users, and client groups in a healthcare perspective, the term 'additional needs' not only encompasses the area of impairment to learning, but also of physical difficulties and conditions that can often result in challenging behaviours.

As practitioners, we may sometimes find the actions of an individual service user particularly difficult or hard to cope with. Whilst we appreciate that this is part of the job, we do need to develop an approach that is not only appropriately responsive, but underpinned by our own professional sense of ethical practice and inclusive working. As student practitioners, you are preparing to work in a sector where you will be in daily contact with individuals who will need support with activities of daily living. Such work takes resilience matched with a knowledgeable appreciation of the difficulties that can present themselves in a number of different, yet commonly recognisable areas.

Disabilities

The Equality Act 2010 defines a disabled person as someone who has 'a physical or mental impairment which has a substantial and long-term adverse effect on his or her ability to carry out normal day-to-day activities'.

It is the effect on their ability to carry out normal day-to-day activities that should be considered. To be defined as a disability, the effect must be long term and substantial. A common misperception is that only disabled people are protected in law; however, the Equality Act enshrines nine protected characteristics (see Table 10.1) for a vast range of individuals belonging to groups who have traditionally been subjected to discriminatory behaviour. Do you know them?

Table 10.1   The protected characteristics

Age
Disability
Gender reassignment
Marriage and civil partnership
Pregnancy and maternity
Race
Religion or belief
Sex
Sexual orientation

SEN and disability

An individual who has an impairment in learning is not by default considered to be disabled. The definition of SEN includes many, but not necessarily all, disabled children:

- A disabled child has SEN if they have a disability and need special educational provision to be made for them to be able to access the education that is available locally.
- The largest group of pupils who may be disabled but do not have SEN are likely to be those with a range of medical conditions – for example, those with severe asthma, arthritis or diabetes may not have SEN but may have rights under the Equality Act.

Similarly, not all children with SEN will be defined as having a disability under the Equality Act:

- Many of the pupils who have SEN or who are at School Action Plus will count as disabled.
- Some children whose emotional and behavioral difficulties have their origins in social or domestic circumstances are identified as having SEN, but may fall outside the definition of disability in the Equality Act.

However, those with a mental health condition are likely to be included where their impairment has a substantial and long-term adverse effect on their ability to carry out normal day-to-day activities.

Disability and the medical model vs. the social model

The discussion around how best to support someone with additional needs has centred traditionally on the conflict between the medical and social model approaches. The medical model views the individual's disability as the root problem, which does not concern anyone other than the individual affected. For example, if a wheelchair user cannot get into a building because of some steps, this model would suggest that this is because of the wheelchair, rather than the steps. However, the social model of disability would see the steps as a barrier, drawing on the idea that it is society that disables people, through designing everything to meet the needs of people who are not disabled. The social model argues that there is a great deal that society can do to reduce and remove disabling barriers, and this is the responsibility of society, rather than the person with the disability.

Genetic research

There are currently two main methodologies for genetic research into psychological functioning: quantitative genetics and molecular genetics.

Quantitative genetics is based on quantifying how genetic and non-genetic factors, such as the surrounding environment, determine the consistent occurrence of particular traits or disorders within groups of people. This approach mainly uses studies which focus closely on the relative influence of the aforementioned factors on human development. The general principle of this methodology is that variation in traits is caused by the cumulative, small effects of many genes, combined with environmental factors.

Studies using quantitative genetics have found major interplay between the two factors, and as such, suggest that disorders cannot be exclusively attributed to either.

Molecular genetics looks at how genes transferred from generation to generation determine an individual's susceptibility to particular mental and physical ailments. Sequencing of the human genome seems likely to advance the discovery of susceptibility genes associated with heritable features, but behavioural geneticist Michael Rutter (2007), has warned it would be misleading to suggest we will soon be able to judge a person's susceptibility from birth. There are a limited number of disorders, such as schizophrenia and autism, for which genetic factors account for much of variance in population – more than 70%. However, there is no single 'autism gene', and identifying specific genes related to individual disorders remains difficult.

Further studies have therefore tried to locate a more definitive causal factor. Benard's 1991 book *Fostering Resiliency in Kids* found that half to two-thirds of children growing up with environmental contributors to BESD were eventually able to adapt to normal behaviour. Her data sample included populations of:

- Children with mentally ill, alcoholic, abusive, or criminally involved parents
- Children growing up in war-torn or economically depressed regions

---

Go Further 10.1

You can read Benard's research as a free pdf at www.wested.org/wp-content/files_mf/1373568312resource93.pdf

---

Autism

Autism is a lifelong developmental disability that affects how a person communicates with, and relates to, other people. It also affects how they make sense of the world around them.

This condition is called a spectrum, as the symptoms are measured against levels of severity. Individuals on the autism spectrum experience difficulties in social interaction and communication, and may have rigid and repetitive ways of thinking and behaving. These behaviours are thought to be underpinned by difficulties in both the flexible generation of ideas and the understanding of other people's thoughts and feelings. There is, however, much variation in the way that children and young people with autism show these different behaviours.

Autism is a developmental condition and the presentation in any individual will change with age, with some children experiencing periods of rapid improvement and others stasis, or plateauing of development. Low self-esteem, failure at tasks, social isolation and irrational thoughts are common difficulties for people with autism, and can contribute to the development of mental health disorders. Children on the autism spectrum may also have a reduced awareness of their own emotional states, meaning that they are less able to plan to avoid stress.

Autism has a strong genetic component, although it is now recognised that this consists of both heritable and sporadic (non-inherited) forms. Until recently, many children with autism were not diagnosed until four or five years of age, and even later for some children with Asperger syndrome or those with good language skills and of average or above-average ability (sometimes referred to as 'high functioning autism'). However, progress has been made in the earlier identification of autism, and many children, especially those with a more classic presentation of autism in combination with language delay, are now often identified before the age of five years.

Other factors that research points to as a potential cause are as follows:

- Brain injury in the womb
- Dietary aspects in infancy
- Low brain stimulation in first weeks
- Associated behaviours (copying that of siblings or parents, for instance)

Some of the distinguishing features of autism are outlined next to help you understand the different way in which people with autism may behave and think.

Monotropism vs. polytropism

The terms 'monotropism' and 'polytropism' refer to the ability to shift and share attention, as seen in Figure 10.1. The polytropic mind can multitask and tends to put a moderate amount of attention into many areas of interest. People with autism are more likely to be monotropic. This means an intense focus on something of interest, and the reduced ability to switch quickly from one task to another.

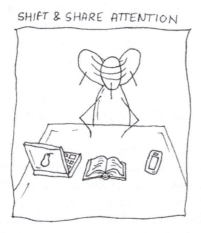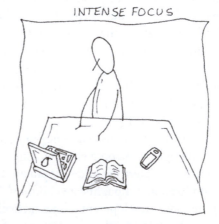

Figure 10.1   Polytropic and monotropic

The theory of mind

Sometimes called 'mentalising' or 'mindreading', the theory of mind (often abbreviated to 'ToM') describes the social ability to understand the motives, intentions and beliefs of others, and to see something from another's point of view – even when that perspective is different from our own. Simon Baron-Cohen has been one of the leading researchers involved in ToM. He explains:

> In my early work, I explored the theory that children with autism spectrum conditions are delayed in developing a theory of mind (ToM): the ability to put oneself into someone else's shoes, to imagine their thoughts and feelings … We not only make sense of another person's behaviour (… Why did their eyes move left?), but we also imagine whole set of mental states (they have seen something of interest, they know something or want something) and we can predict what they might do next … [This] theory proposes that children with autism and Asperger's syndrome are delayed in the development of ToM. (Baron-Cohen, 1997a: 113)

The Sally–Anne test is a psychological test used to measure social cognitive ability to attribute false beliefs to others (see Figure 10.2). The test involves two dolls, 'Sally' and 'Anne'. Sally has a basket. Anne has a box. Sally puts a ball in her basket and then leaves the scene. While Sally is away and cannot watch, Anne takes the ball out of Sally's basket and puts it into her box. Sally then returns, and the child is asked where she/he thinks she will look for her ball. Children are said to 'pass' the test if they understand that Sally will most likely look inside her basket before realising that her ball isn't there. Children under the age of four, along with most autistic children (of older ages), will answer, 'Anne's box', seemingly unaware that Sally does not know her ball has been moved.

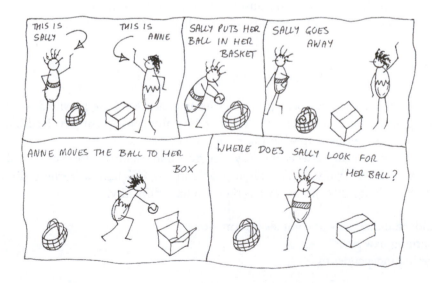

Figure 10.2   Sally and Anne (taken from a description by Baron-Cohen, 1997)

Central coherence theory

People on the autism spectrum tend to focus in on detail and may have difficulty understanding the 'bigger picture'. Children with developing minds will tend to seek out context, so have a strong central coherence often described as the ability to understand surrounding contexts or see 'the bigger picture' (Frith, 1989). Baron-Cohen (1997b, 2008) captured the essence of this theory by suggesting that people on the autistic spectrum have problems in integrating information to make a coherent, global picture. Instead they will often focus on the small, local details in a scene. The neurotypical mind, with strong central coherence, is more likely to attend to the gist, rather than the nitty-gritty.

Some theorists suggest that people with autism process faces and, therefore, emotions in unconventional ways. For example, some individuals with autism can easily recognise faces upside down – a task that neurotypical individuals find more difficult. This suggests that people with autism use individual features of the face to recognise people and emotions, rather than the whole face. These differences in facial processing may lead to difficulties in recognising emotions, and individuals may confuse the feelings of others. This confusion is not only limited to facial expression, and may apply to other forms of communication, such as body language.

The effect of colour

Colour can be an important factor in affecting the mood of a child with autism. Different colour schemes may have a calming, stimulating, or even disturbing effect on those with autism. Studies have found that certain colour schemes are preferred by service users and carers. Subdued or pastel colours mixed with grey, colours in blue or green hue and colours in solid, unpatterned blocks were preferential. Noise reduction strategies can be useful for some individuals on the autism spectrum. In terms of practice, alterations to the environment may go a long way to address challenging behaviours.

LEARNING DIFFICULTIES

Over time, thinkers, researchers, psychologists and theorists have provided many reasons for poor achievement. The term 'learning difficulty' consequently evolved. There is also a lack of consensus as to what this term actually means.

A learning difficulty affects the way a person understands information and how they communicate. Around 1.5 million people in the UK have a learning difficulty (MentalHealth.org, 2017). This means they can have difficulty:

- understanding new or complex information
- learning new skills
- coping independently

In the UK, the terms *profound*, *severe*, *moderate* and *mild* have been used to describe people with learning disabilities, but there are no clear dividing lines between the groups. Furthermore, there is no clear cut-off point between people with mild learning disabilities and the general population, and you may hear the term *borderline learning disability* being used. In the past, a diagnosis of a learning disability and understanding of a person's needs was based on IQ scores; today the importance of a holistic approach is recognised, and IQ testing forms only one small part of assessing someone's strengths and needs. Table 10.2 identifies each category in more detail.

Table 10.2   Categories of learning difficulty

Profound intellectual and multiple disabilities	This refers to people with a profound intellectual disability (an IQ of less than 20) and in addition they may have other disabilities such as visual, hearing or movement impairments, or they may have autism or epilepsy. People in this category have the highest levels of care needs in our communities
Severe learning disability	This refers to people with an IQ of between 20 and 35. Many need a high level of support with everyday activities, but they may be able to look after some if not all their own personal care needs
Moderate learning disability	This refers to people with an IQ of 35 to 50. They are likely to have some language skills, which means they can communicate about their day-to-day needs and wishes. Some people may need more support caring for themselves, but many will be able to carry out day to day tasks
Mild learning disability	This refers to people with an IQ of 50 to 70. They are usually able to hold a conversation and communicate most of their needs and wishes. They may need some support to understand abstract or complex ideas. People are often independent in caring for themselves and doing many everyday tasks

Learning disability and the medical model vs. the social model

As discussed earlier, the social and medical models have had a profound influence on society's approaches to inclusion and care of the vulnerable. Here we will consider them in relation to learning difficulties more specifically.

The medical model asserts that an individual's level of ability is the main determining cause of low attainment. It looks at learning difficulties as an individual issue so, someone struggling to keep up with their peers may be deemed 'slow', without considering the wider context of their environment. In more general terms, this model places the onus on how a disability impairs an individual and makes them 'different' from the rest of society, rather than looking at surrounding factors that define this. It is the physical impairment (or in the case of identifying a learning difficulty) that makes the person disabled, rather than the limitations of the world in which they live.

By contrast, the social model focuses on the effects of the surrounding environment on an individual. When taking the perspective of this model, difficulties with learning, such as those experienced by children identified as having a form of mild learning difficulty, are due to shortcomings in support from the educational environment or at home. In contrast to the medical model, this viewpoint considers circumstances to be failing the child and as such emphasises the need for organisational change. In a wider context, it looks at how people's surrounding environments and society's negative attitudes, exclusions and barriers can exacerbate impairments and turn them into disabilities.

In their 2005 book *Moderate Learning Difficulties and the Future of Inclusion* Narcie Kelly and Brahm Norwich described a 'false opposition' between the two models. They state that there is neither a 'right' nor 'wrong' model to follow, and the two are not mutually exclusive. As each position has strengths and weaknesses, they need to complement one another and be applied to circumstances. Using only one of the two models for teaching individuals with learning difficulties can result in limitations. For example:

- Encouraging low expectations by only focusing on the individual's difficulties in the medical model.
- Failing to account for diversity by focusing only on structures and practice in social model.

Practitioners must understand and be mindful of both approaches, taking account of all factors when evaluating anyone. How this is achieved in practice essentially comes down to the use of the practitioner's own reflective thinking and observations. Making reasonable adjustments to access and in providing one-to-one support are all practical measures commonly pursued to ensure a basic but effective form of inclusion.

Dyslexia

Dyslexia is a language processing disorder that can hinder reading, writing, spelling and sometimes even speaking. Dyslexia is not a sign of poor intelligence or laziness. The Rose Report (Rose, 2009) said dyslexic difficulties 'are best thought of as existing on a continuum from mild to severe, rather than forming a discrete category'. While it stated there was no sharp dividing line of having or not having dyslexia, it defined three characteristic features:

[1] Phonological awareness
   This is the ability to hear and analyse the sounds within words. It is understood to be the key skill required for learning phonics and acquiring the alphabetic principle.
[2] Verbal memory
   Verbal memory difficulties may give the impression that a pupil has not been paying attention, and include an inability to recall verbal instructions, failing to respond or responding slowly to questions. Issues with note taking, essay planning and self-organisation can be seriously troublesome for older pupils with greater than usual difficulties in verbal memory.
[3] Verbal processing speed
   This is the time it takes to process familiar verbal information, such as letters and digits. In your practice, this could involve the provision of additional time to assimilate information and complete tasks.

Behavioral, emotional and social difficulties (BESD) and social, emotional and mental health (SEMH) difficulties

Challenging behaviour is that which does not follow a socially and cultural normative pattern and is both complex and challenging in many ways. Behavioural, emotional and social difficulties (BESD) and social, emotional and mental health difficulties (SEMH) are umbrella terms to describe a range of complex and chronic difficulties experienced by many individuals. Some commonly recognised traits include the following:

- Being withdrawn or isolated
- Displaying a disruptive and disturbing nature
- Being hyperactive and lacking concentration
- Having immature social skills
- Presenting challenging behaviours arising from other complex special needs

The frequency, intensity and duration of such behaviour is of a much higher level and the need for additional support in developing various emotional competencies is much more crucial to social and emotional development in an individual. For these reasons, behavioral disorders are judged to be more challenging for the practitioner to deal with. However, as you get to know your service user, you will gain a better understanding of their triggers to challenging behaviours and their particular preferences.

Current approaches recognise a complex relationship between environmental and genetic factors. In *Genes and Behaviour: Nature–Nurture Interplay Explained* (2006), Sir Michael Rutter argues that environmental factors will influence a genetic predisposition towards behavioral problems, either by increasing or decreasing its effects. In the 1960s, there was broad acceptance of the lasting and irreversible effects of early childhood experiences. There was also a consensus that social disadvantage was a major cause of BESD. During the 1980s, research found that the same or similar environmental factors could lead to a range of outcomes between various individual cases. As we moved away from this outlook the nature of behavioural disorders was explored in much greater depth, and thus consideration was given to individual competence and how practice could support people's autonomy.

Goleman (1996) identified five emotional competencies, which are of arguable significance to the development of social and emotional skills:

[1] Awareness of self and others. Essentially, this is an appreciation of the impact on each other's feelings as well as our own.
[2] Mood management. The control of impulses and anger.
[3] Self-motivation. Working towards specified goals, despite setbacks and occasional surmountable barriers.
[4] Empathy. The ability to see things from other people's perspectives and to understand resultant associated emotions both cognitively and affectively.
[5] Relationship management. The ability to cooperate with others when necessary and to form friendship, whilst resolving conflicts appropriately.

Therefore, support mechanisms must therefore be created and put in place to facilitate the development of each competency, and these should address the barriers that result from challenging behaviour. The effectiveness of individual strategies that are used is therefore assessable against best practice measures, and can be adjusted according to the circumstances at any given point. Given the shifting nature of attitudes towards behavioral disorders over time, it is important that we consider a couple of the more prominent disorders that fall into the BESD category to enhance our own professional understanding of the approaches used to enable support.

Attention deficit hyperactivity disorder (ADHD)

Attention deficit hyperactivity disorder (ADHD) describes the behaviours displayed by some children who are extremely restless and energetic. These children are often impatient and find it difficult to filter out other things going on around them. Typically, they will have an incredibly short attention span and find it difficult to concentrate on specific tasks. ADHD is the most common childhood-onset behavioural disorder, and it affects around 4% of children in the UK (AA-DD UK, 2017). Research by Nøvik et al. (2006) suggests that it is approximately three times more common in boys than in girls, although recent research suggests that girls express ADHD differently (NICE, 2016).

Methylphenidate (trade name Ritalin) is widely prescribed to raise chronically low levels of dopamine activity in people with ADHD. In studies of its effects, 80% of children were able to improve their focus, attention span and impulse control.

However, some participants reported side effects, such as:

- Reduced appetite and weight loss
- Mild sleep disturbance
- Headaches

Professionals recommend that Ritalin is used only to treat children older than 6 years of age, and that treatment should be halted periodically to assess its impact.

Model of anger

This model can help practitioners to raise awareness about the processes of anger with service users using social learning theory. Visual representations such as 'the match',

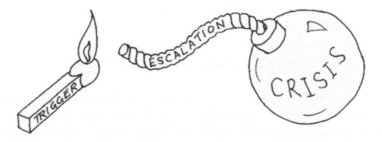

Figure 10.3   Model of anger

'the fuse' and 'the explosion' (Figure 10.3) help people to understand responses to anger by mapping an anger model to pictures. In this case, the match represents the anger trigger, the fuse represents escalation and the explosion represents the crisis phase.

> ## Go Further 10.2
>
> Read this chapter – www.advanced-training.org.uk/ – to enhance your understanding of anger triggers and how to manage them.

Oppositional defiant disorder (ODD)

Oppositional defiant disorder (ODD) is a psychiatric disorder. It is typically characterised by hostile behaviour towards figures of authority – and of a far more severe nature than what can usually be expected from normal childhood behaviour.

Typical behaviours will last over six months and will include:

- Swearing or use of obscene language
- Deliberately annoys other pupils or staff at school
- Child often angry and resentful
- Argumentative nature
- Child is often spiteful or vindictive
- Problems with losing temper
- Refusal to work or follow instructions
- Easy to offend or becomes oversensitive

The causes of oppositional defiant disorder are poorly understood but influence from parents is thought to be a contributing factor. Other factors may include:

- The environment in which a child is brought up, including lack of supervision, poor quality of housing or instability in the family
- A genetic predisposition may be present
- The nature of the child or adolescent such as 'touchiness' or spitefulness will increase the chances of developing ODD

Ensuring a comfortable environment and gaining a greater understanding of the traits that express themselves through ODD is crucial to accommodating to it. An example would be to adjust your approach so that the service user feels less threatened and oppressed within your environment.

PHYSICAL DIFFICULTIES

Physical disability pertains to **total** or **partial loss** of a person's bodily functions (e.g., walking, gross motor skills, bladder control etc.) and **total** or **partial loss** of a part of the body (e.g., an amputation).

Examples of physical disability include:

- Cerebral palsy
- Muscular dystrophy
- Acquired brain injury
- Cerebral vascular event (stroke)
- Alzheimer's disease and vascular dementia

There are many kinds of disability and a wide variety of situations which people experience:

- The disability may exist from birth or be acquired later in life.
- A person may have one disability or a number of disabilities.
- A person may be treated as having a disability when in fact he or she does not.
- A person's disability may be apparent, such as loss of a limb; or hidden, such as epilepsy or deafness.
- Disability may be more (or less) severe in its impact.
- People with the same disability are as likely as anyone else to have different abilities.
- Situations where a brain injury has occurred since birth.

Historically, disabled people have been viewed with a variety of emotions including suspicion, ridicule and pity. Until recently, they have been excluded almost completely from all aspects of community life. Our culture is full of disablist language and imagery which has the effect of maintaining the traditional fears and prejudices which surround impairment.

Physical disability and the medical model vs. the social model

Many people think that disability is caused by an individual's health condition or impairment (the medical model). In this view, one might say that by fixing their body, disabled people will be able to participate in society just like everyone else. The social model of disability, on the other hand, suggests that disability is created by barriers in society itself, which generally fall into three categories:

- **The environment** – including inaccessible buildings and services
- **People's attitudes** – stereotyping, discrimination and prejudice
- **Organisations** – inflexible policies, practices and procedures.

There are a variety of physical disabilities that impact on the approaches you will have to take in supporting those with impairments such as traumatic brain injury.

Traumatic brain injury

Traumatic brain injury is the result of things happening outside of the body – such as an accident to the head in a car or bike accident. Non-traumatic brain injury is the result of happenings inside the head, such as a tumour or stroke. Brain injuries, howsoever caused, can lead to impairments and challenging behaviours such as:

- Cognitive (which is just a more technical way of describing some of the processes that go on in our head): Limited attention span, trouble remembering things, difficulties processing information.
- Emotions and behaviour: Self-esteem, feelings of being behind, difficulties controlling emotions, distractedness, impatience, frustrations, trouble socialising with other children.
- Physical: Pain or discomfort, lack of access to parts of the school, restrictions to getting involved in PE, tiredness/fatigue, sleep disruption, seizures.

DEMENTIA

Dementia is a cluster of symptoms based on memory loss. There are several different causes, the most common being Alzheimer's disease. Alzheimer's disease is the build-up of proteins in the brain which then form structures called 'plaques' and 'tangles' (Andrews, 2015). The loss of connections between nerve cells breaks the message transmitting ability, and leads to the death of nerve cells and loss of brain tissue. The next most prevalent cause is vascular dementia, which is due to brain cell death by lack of oxygen, which might be caused by a stroke or mini-stroke (transient ischaemic attack or TIA). The blood vessels become blocked or clogged by cholesterol plaques or blood clots. Vascular dementia is characterised by a 'stepping down' of the sufferer's cognitive ability rather than the steady decline of Alzheimer's. The third main cause of dementia is Lewy bodies. Lewy body dementia (DLB) shares symptoms with Alzheimer's and with Parkinson's disease, and is caused by Tau protein build-up within nerve cells. In the early stages of the disease the sufferer may experience visual or auditory hallucinations. They also have 'good' days and 'bad' days, which may in fact be good/bad weeks. DLB is progressive and the person slowly declines over time.

It is useful to understand that it is not just those of an older age who develop dementia. There is a small but increasing number of young people (early onset) who develop this; the Alzheimer's Society (2015) suggests 42,000 or 5% of those with dementia are young people. It is likely to be hereditary (familial Alzheimer's) or, in some cases, caused through substance misuse (mainly alcohol). However, this may be reversed with abstinence and a good diet rich in thiamine.

📖 Scenario 10.2

Jewels Ford, an adult social worker, visited Mrs Oliver who is an inpatient on an NHS trust ward, as part of her discharge planning. The nursing notes were indecisive in terms of diagnosis; the nurses considered that she had had a fall while suffering a urinary tract infection (UTI). However, Mrs Oliver's daughter gave a narrative which might suggest she was suffering from dementia.

Why would the nursing staff decide that a UTI is most likely cause of the fall and why do you think her daughter would consider her mother had dementia?

What are the similarities and differences between these two diagnosis?

Challenging behaviour and dementia

Behaviour is a form of communication and body language is as eloquent as the spoken word. Behaviour is culturally mediated (see Chapter 11, Introduction to Mental Health and Wellbeing for further detail) and each culture has different behavioural expectations. Common behaviour for sufferers of dementia is 'wandering' and 'rummaging'; clearly the person is engaged in some activity which is meaningful to them. It is unusual for dementia sufferers to be violent, unless they feel they are being threatened.

It is important that care staff, family and friends explain clearly and in a language the person understands any activity they wish them to participate in, and that consent is obtained before any intervention takes place (see Chapter 7, Essential Skills for Care, for further details about consent). Some clients are subject to Deprivation of Liberty Orders (DoLs) and this requires an intervention under the Mental Capacity Act 2005 as it must be in the person's best interest, and extra safeguards must be in place before restraint can be used. At least six assessments must take place before the local authority can give authorisation. The person subject to DoL must have a 'relevant person's representative' and have access to an Independent Mental Capacity Advocate (IMCA).

PROFESSIONAL APPROACHES TO ADDITIONAL NEEDS AND CHALLENGING BEHAVIOURS

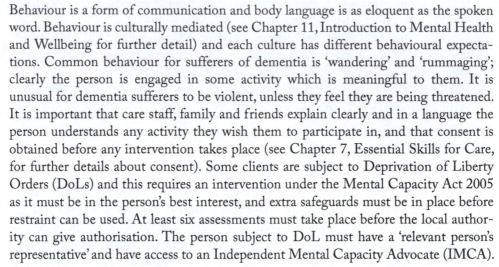

Abrams (2010) defines prejudice as 'bias which devalues people because of their perceived membership of a social group'. Prejudice ultimately involves stereotyping and prejudging people. A stereotype is a highly simplified idea held about a group. When we create a stereotypical concept, we make shortcuts in our thinking which, in some situations, can be damaging. For clients and service users, their sense of identity can be affected if they are at the receiving end of negative attitudes towards themselves, and/or the group to which they belong. They may feel that certain options are not available or open to them.

So, is it possible to stop prejudicial views? Abrams (2010) found in research that the more contact there is with people from other groups and cultures and the more understanding there is, the more likely prejudice and discrimination will be reduced. There is an on-going need for those working with the vocational sector to be involved in training that is high quality and relevant to the sector. Training, however, is not enough on its own, as there are personal qualities and competencies that those working within the sector need. We should ultimately recognise that inclusion is about fostering the individual needs of each person and offering an equal opportunity to reach their potential. Inclusion and inclusive practice are requirements that support the individual needs of all disabled people, and break down barriers to segregation and exclusion.

There are issues to be addressed before full inclusion becomes a reality and inclusion is the right of all individuals, and these issues need consideration by all practitioners. All staff should take a leadership role within their workplace to discuss and find measures to mitigate the following:

- Policies (both local and nation) are often ineffective
- Training is not provided for all grades
- Pay amongst practitioners varies greatly depending on sector
- Profile of workers needs to be improved in many cases
- Access to resources needs to be widened
- More focus on 'needs-led' provision as opposed to 'budget-led' provision
- Funding issues need to be addressed

You can read more on leadership skills in Chapter 4, Leadership and Teamwork.

So, what then is good practice? In theory, it is the removal of barriers, the promotion of diversity, the creation of equal opportunities and the challenging of discrimination. We have a duty not to discriminate against people with disabilities and to make reasonable adjustments where required to support individuals with additional needs. These include accommodation and access, alongside other additional adjustments to enable access to opportunities for all.

Discrimination

Discrimination is failing to take reasonable steps to ensure you do not place a disabled person at a 'substantial disadvantage'. Key to any student practitioner's understanding and appreciation of how to tackle discrimination, is to understand that to treat someone differently as a result of their difference is not automatically a negative act.

Occasionally, a person will be discriminated against in favour of another, in which case we are deemed to be taking what is often referred to as 'positive discrimination' or in most cases, 'positive action'. The purpose of positive action is to allow disadvantaged people the same rights and opportunities as advantaged people.

Health and social care settings adhere to the stipulations laid down in the Equality Act 2010, translating this into practice, ever mindful however, that our day-to-day work with vulnerable client groups and service users necessitates the requirement to maintain awareness and understanding of how discrimination can manifest itself. Sometimes this is in the form of the most basic behaviours, which can carry substantial impacts with service users, no matter how harmless our approaches seem to us as practitioners.

Safeguarding

The Care Act 2012 sets out the clear legal frameworks for each local authority and the need for multi-agency adult safeguarding boards. The board must review cases where abuse is suspected and there is concern that the local authority has not responded appropriately.

Abuse can be neglect, physical, mental, financial, sexual, domestic, discriminatory or organisational. It is incumbent upon you as a health and social care worker to undertake safeguarding training, and to familiarise yourself with your organisation's policies and procedures in order to know where to turn if you witness or suspect abuse. Further information on safeguarding is found in Chapter 12, Protecting Children and Vulnerable Adults.

CHAPTER SUMMARY

- The number of conditions we have considered in this chapter is by no means an exhaustive list.
- We should not overlook the fact that the debate around causes and impacts of a variety of additional needs and challenging behaviours will continue to develop, creating an ever-changing perception of the barriers that people face, in turn fuelling changes in the way that we as practitioners conduct our duties.
- However, this chapter's aim has been to provide you with a starting point for your professional practice and to get you to think deeper about how you can work with service users, patients and families in the best possible way and in line with their needs, regardless of their abilities and conditions.
- Your approaches in your healthcare practice will be shaped, morphed and informed further through ongoing reflective exercises, based upon the familiarity you will have with individual client groups during the course of your practice.
- Observing matters from the perspective of the service user remains key to addressing any barriers to opportunity and progress that you may encounter, as ultimately you are there to provide a service to support, enable and fulfil the needs of those who are less advantaged than ourselves.

FURTHER READING

You can deepen your knowledge and understanding of additional needs and challenging behaviours by visiting these websites and reading the recommended texts

Websites

- Alzheimer's Society: www.alzhiemers.org.uk
- Advanced training materials for a range of learning and behavioural difficulties: www.advanced-training.org.uk
- The National Autistic Society: www.autism.org.uk

Texts

- Abrams, D. (2010) *Processes of Prejudice: Theory, Evidence and Intervention.* Available at: www.equalityhumanrights.com/en/publication-download/research-report-56-processes-prejudice-theory-evidence-and-intervention (accessed 14 March 2017).
- Andrews, J. (2015) *Dementia: The One-Stop Guide: Practical Advice for Families, Professionals, and People Living with Dementia and Alzheimer's Disease.* London: Profile.
- Baron-Cohen, S. (1997) *Mindblindness: An Essay on Autism and the Theory of Mind* (Learning, Development and Conceptual Change Series). Cambridge, MA: MIT Press.

- Baron-Cohen, S. (2008) *Autism and Asperger Syndrome (The Facts)*. Oxford: Oxford University Press.
- Daley, G. (2008) *Anger: A Solution Focussed Approach for Young People*. Optimus Education.
- Frith, U. (1989) *Autism: Explaining the Enigma*. Oxford: Blackwell.
- Goleman, D. (2006) *Emotional Intelligence: Why It Can Matter More Than IQ* (10th Anniversary edition). London: Bantam.
- Kelly, N. and Norwich, B. (2004) *Moderate Learning Difficulties and the Future of Inclusion*. Abingdon: Routledge/Falmer.
- Northway, R. and Jenkins, R. (2017) *Safeguarding Adults in Nursing Practice* (2nd edn) (Transforming Nursing Practice Series). London: Sage.

REFERENCES

AA-DD UK (2107) *What is ADHD?* [online]. Available at: aadduk.org (accessed 26 March 2017).

Abrams, D. (2010) *Processes of Prejudice: Theory, Evidence and Intervention*. Available at: www.equalityhumanrights.com/en/publication-download/research-report-56-processes-prejudice-theory-evidence-and-intervention (accessed 19 June 2017).

Alzheimer's Society (2015) *Factsheet 440: What is Young-onset Dementia?* [online]. Available at: www.alzheimers.org.uk/site/scripts/download_info.php?downloadID=1104 (accessed 27 March 2017).

Andrews, J. (2015) *Dementia: The One-Stop Guide. Practical advice for families, professionals, and people living with dementia and Alzheimer's disease*. London: Profile.

Benard, B. (1991) *Fostering Resiliency in Kids*. Available at: www.wested.org/wp-content/files_mf/1373568312resource93.pdf (accessed 27 March 2017).

Baron-Cohen, S. (1997a) *Mindblindness: An Essay on Autism and the Theory of Mind* (Learning, Development and Conceptual Change Series). Cambridge, MA: MIT Press.

Baron-Cohen, S. (1997b) *Theories of the Autistic Mind*. Available at: www.neuroscience.cam.ac.uk/publications/download.php?id=40524 (accessed 10 April 2017).

Baron-Cohen, S. (2008) *Autism and Asperger Syndrome (The Facts)*. Oxford: Oxford University Press.

Frith, U. (1989) *Autism: Explaining the Enigma*. Blackwell: Oxford

Goleman, D. (1996) *Emotional Intelligence: Why It Can Matter More Than IQ*. London: Bloomsbury [10th Anniversary edition, Bantam, 2006].

Kelly, N. and Norwich, B. (2005) *Moderate Learning Difficulties and the Future of Inclusion*. Abingdon: Routledge/Falmer.

MentalHealth.org (2017) *Learning Disability Statistics* [online]. Available at: www.mentalhealth.org.uk/learning-disabilities/help-information/learning-disability-statistics- (accessed 24 March 2017).

NICE (National Institute for Health and Care Excellence) (2016) *Attention Deficit Hyperactivity Disorder: Diagnosis and Management*. Clinical Guideline (CG) 72 [online]. Available at: www.nice.org.uk/guidance/cg72 (accessed 27 March 2017).

Nøvik, T.S., Hervas, A., Ralston, S.J., Dalsgaard, S., Rodrigues Pereira, R. and Lorenzo, M.J. (2006) Influence of gender on attention-deficit/hyperactivity disorder in Europe. *European Child Adolescence Psychiatry*, 15(Suppl. 1): I15–24.

Rose, J. (2009) *Independent Review of the Primary Curriculum: Final Report*. Available at: www.educationengland.org.uk/documents/pdfs/2009-IRPC-final-report.pdf (accessed 10 April 2017).

Rutter, M. (2006) *Genes and Behaviour: Nature–Nurture Interplay Explained*. Oxford: Wiley Blackwell.

Rutter, M. (2007) Gene–environment interdependence. *Developmental Science Journal*, 10(1): 12–18.

11

INTRODUCTION TO MENTAL HEALTH AND WELLBEING

Gillian Rowe

St Mary's of Bethlehem hospital was described in 1450 by the Lord Mayor of London as a place where may 'be found many men that be fallen out of their wit. And full honestly they be kept in that place; and some be restored onto their wit and health again. And some be abiding therein for ever.'

This chapter is an introduction to mental health and wellbeing. You will consider what factors make us think that someone is unwell and how we categorise ailments, and then we will examine how those categorisations can lead to people being labelled. We live in a multicultural society and, as has been considered in other chapters, people from other ethnicities are overrepresented within the mental healthcare system and this will be considered. Historically, mental health sufferers have been stigmatised as lacking moral fibre and the quote by the Lord Mayor of London (1450) shows how historically there was no real treatment other than containment. While we still have secure wards, medical interventions and therapies are preferred options, although we still have a long way to go in combating the stigma that is attached to poor mental health.

📌 Glossary

- **Depot injections** Long-acting medications
- **Interventions** Any treatment
- **Sectioning** Detention under one of the sections of the Mental Health Act 1983, 2007
- **Stigma** A negative attitude towards mental health sufferers

INTRODUCTION AND DEFINITIONS

The current model of mental health considers that mental disorders are disorders of brain circuits caused by developmental processes shaped through a complex interplay of genetics and experience. The word 'mental' is viewed as a negative, but we are mental as well as physical entities, and our mental makeup defines who we are. The World Health Organization define this by stating 'Mental health is the emotional resilience which enables us to enjoy life and to survive pain, disappointment and sadness. It is a positive sense of wellbeing and an underlying belief in our and others dignity and worth' (WHO, 2014). Developing poor mental health is characterised by changes in our thinking, mood and behaviours; this chapter will introduce you to explanations or models of mental health, why mental health is stigmatised, treatment options for sufferers and how we can support ourselves when suffering from stress.

⚙ Activity 11.1

Think for a moment of all the words to describe mental health. Draw two boxes: in one write positive and the other negative words. Positive words might include sane, mentally healthy, and your negative box might include such words as mad, bonkers, loopy etc. Is there a difference between the number of positive and negative words?

What is being mentally healthy? The Mental Health Foundation (2017) says if you can manage all these things, you are mentally healthy:

- make the most of your potential
- cope with life
- play a full part in your family, workplace, community and among friends
- learn
- feel, express and manage a range of positive and negative emotions
- form and maintain good relationships with others
- cope with and manage change and uncertainty

⚙ Activity 11.2

Write your own definition of being mentally healthy in the space below

One of the drawbacks of being mentally unwell is that it has few physical symptoms. Mental health can be explained in terms of behaviours and expressed emotions. What is or is not acceptable behaviour is culturally mediated and Thomas Szasz (1961) argued that mental illness is a metaphor for the 'problems in living', that mental ill health was a myth and that the description 'mental ill health' is a euphemism for behaviours that are socially disapproved of.

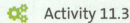

Activity 11.3

Look up the disease 'drapetomania'. Now also consider 'oppositional defiant disorder'. Do you think they are mental health disorders?

CATEGORISING MENTAL HEALTH

The lack of a universally agreed cut-off point between normal behaviour and behaviour associated with mental illness means that a diagnosis is usually made after a recognition of personal distress, either by the person or by the person's family/friends. The *Diagnostic and Statistical Manual* is a diagnostic handbook created by the American Psychiatric Association. It is the awkward child of the needs of the medical insurance industry for reimbursement and the need of the medical profession to categorise and label signs and symptoms. DSM 1 was published in 1952, it was 145 pages long and contained 106 disorders; the latest iteration is DSM 5 (2013) and is 947 pages long and contains an indeterminate number of disorders (157–300 depending on who you read). The health professions in the UK also use the International Classification of Diseases (ICD), which is hosted by the World Health Organisation (WHO.org). The current iteration is ICD 10 (1990) and ICD 11 is due in 2018. The ICD is not restricted to mental health but identifies all diseases and disorders. DSM 5 also removed the Global Assessment of Function (GAF scale) for assessing people in terms of their ailments and have adopted the WHODAS 2.0 scale. This is based on, and reflects, the assessment of impairment and disability and is separate from diagnostic considerations, its utility being that it can reflect any medical illness, psychiatric illness or comorbid condition.

For many people, the existing systems of categorising illnesses do not relate closely enough to their experiences. Those with enduring complex mental health issues struggle to identify their feelings and emotions with their diagnosis. Recall the explanation of the sick role given in Chapter 8, Applied Health Sciences. Parsons (1951) felt the function of the sick role is necessary to maintain social order, but the reality is more complex. Gabe et al. (2006) discussed the work of Zola (1973), and considered the not-so-obvious question of why a person seeks medical attention. Zola suggested it was as a result of the person's inability to cope with the symptoms, such as when the symptoms begin to impact on a person's ability to get on with their life, work and relationships. Table 11.1 gives some examples of behaviours that have been named or labelled. Jerome Wakefield and Allan Horrwitz (2006) state, 'What makes a medical disorder mental rather than (exclusively) somatic or physical? Psychiatry to some extent depends for its existence as a medical specialty on the distinction between mental and somatic disorders, yet the history of this distinction presents a bewildering array of puzzling judgments, radical shifts, and seemingly arbitrary distinctions.'

Table 11.1   Behaviours associated with mental health issues

Disconnection from reality and detachment from social rules

Self-neglect

Attention-seeking behaviours including self-harm

Loss of inhibition such as inappropriate sexual behaviours

Suicidal ideation

Obsessive–compulsive activities

Voice hearing

Panic attacks

Anxiety

Depression

The main models of mental health

The medical model

In Western medical thinking, the medical model is the prevailing explanation. It considers the body to be an organism that consists of natural functions designed by nature, and illness is the breakdown of some of these functions; this is also considered to be a 'deficit' model, viewed from a biological perspective. It is considered mechanistic, in that the body is described as a machine that fails from time to time. Therefore, any dysfunction of the mind is an ailment that results from a disease process such as a chemical imbalance or physical changes in the brain. The medical model gives names to groups of symptoms and calls them a disease and this gives rise to the notion that people become labelled through the process of diagnosis. Cure rests in the hands of the medical profession who are the knowledge experts and who hold the reins of power in health interactions.

Unwell or disabled people are viewed as deviant or in some way inferior; that their disability places restrictions on their ability to participate in economic activity and so they are burdens on the state.

Arguments against the medical model suggest the model is inflexible and fails to recognise its fallibility. Zigmond (2010) considers that the model has its roots in the

scientific process and it only works when the phenomenum can be quantified and measured. Illich (1976) was a vocal protagonist of the model, citing iatrogenic causes such as
clinical injury, cultural iatrogenesis (the disregard of cultural (lay) health practices) and
the medicalisation of normal human conditions such as sadness, loneliness and bereave-
ment. Psychiatric iatrogenesis includes misdiagnosis, the side effects of psychotropic
medication and the medicalisation of adolescent disaffection.

The social model

The social model offers explanations that are related to the experience of those suffering poor health. It recognises that notions of health are socially created and that
society has a mediating role through such things as the environment, education and
housing. It regards an individual's environment and their health as being intrinsically
linked, especially in terms of the conditions in which we live and work, the food that
we eat and the products that we use. Lang (2001) considers that 'disabled people are
subject to oppression and negative social attitudes, that inevitably undermine their
personhood and their status as full citizens'. Foucault (1973) suggested that modern
medicine is part of a process of regulating and disciplining both individual bodies and
the social body.

The breakdown of traditional community, loss of support by geographic mobility
away from family, and low social economic status are all implicated. This does not
exclude the wealthy and well educated from the model, but makes the point that society
needs to adapt and to adopt more inclusive ways of being.

Arguments against the social model include its inability to find cures or develop
successful treatments to alleviate the symptoms of disease and that the medical model
is scrutinised, transparent and objective (Goldacre, 2008). Table 11.2 explains how
Charli's ailments are explained using both models.

The psychodynamic and cognitive models

The psychodynamic model is premised on the work of Sigmund Freud and the notion
that childhood experiences are crucial in shaping adult personality (McWilliams, 2009).
Whilst much of Freud's work is still contested, there is good evidence that unconscious
processes influence our behaviour (Robinson and Gordon, 2011). Freud's model of the

Table 11.2   Charli's ailments

Charli is suffering from myalgia encephalomyelitis (ME), this is episodic and Charli has good days
and bad days

Charli also suffers from depression and poor self-efficacy; on bad days, Charli needs a carer to
support the activities of daily living

On good days, Charli feels well enough to go to work but does not have a job that allows this
flexibility

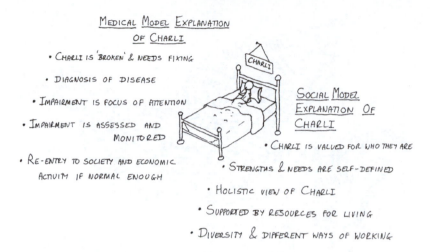

MEDICAL MODEL EXPLANATION
OF CHARLI

• CHARLI IS 'BROKEN' & NEEDS FIXING

• DIAGNOSIS OF DISEASE

• IMPAIRMENT IS FOCUS OF ATTENTION

• IMPAIRMENT IS ASSESSED AND
MONITORED

• RE-ENTRY TO SOCIETY AND ECONOMIC
ACTIVITY IF NORMAL ENOUGH

CHARLI

SOCIAL MODEL
EXPLANATION OF
CHARLI

• CHARLI IS VALUED FOR WHO THEY ARE

• STRENGTHS & NEEDS ARE SELF-DEFINED

• HOLISTIC VIEW OF CHARLI

• SUPPORTED BY RESOURCES FOR LIVING

• DIVERSITY & DIFFERENT WAYS OF WORKING

Figure 11.1   Medical and social models of disability

mind has withstood the test of time (id, ego and super ego) and psychodynamic analysts focus on ego defence mechanisms when working with clients suffering anxiety. The cognitive model is premised on the notion that dysfunctional thinking can lead to poor mental health. It has strong links with the work of Jean Piaget and Edward Tolman and this approach is considered analogous to the working of a computer's central processing systems (Atkinson and Shiffrin, 1968). Cognitive behavioural therapy is one of the practical applications of this theory to mitigate established patterns of thinking habits such as negative self-censure or harsh self-criticism.

The spiritual model

The spiritual model considers how belief in 'something greater than ourselves' can support people with poor mental health. For a long time, holding a religious belief was considered to be a symptom of mental illness (religious mania, voice hearing); certainly Freud linked religion with neurosis. However, Turbott (1996) stated that a rapprochement between religion and psychiatry was essential for psychiatric practice to be effective. Whilst spirituality is a global phenomenon, it does not need to be anchored into any particular religious belief or tradition, whereas religious belief is in many ways 'institutionalised' spirituality with a specific set of rituals. Non-religious people often experience a spiritual void in their lives and seek answers to give hope and peace in their mind. Religious places provide a calm space and spiritual advisors who can give positive support; often they will offer this to both believers and non-believers alike. Encouraging people to explore what is important to them spiritually can be a valuable self-help strategy, and give meaning and direction to someone who feels lost.

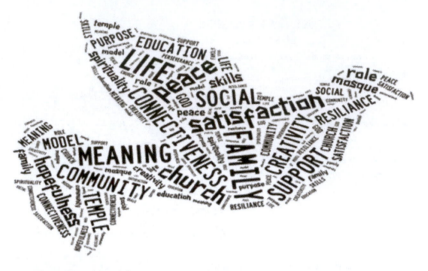

Figure 11.2   The spiritual model

The biopsychosocial model

Devised by cardiologists George Engel and John Romano in 1977, as a result of their awareness that cardiovascular disease is the result of not just biology but sociocultural and psychological influences too, this model incorporates features of the medical, social and psychological models. It is considered both scientific and humanistic. Engel (1977)

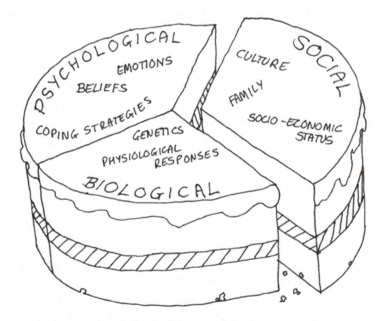

Figure 11.3   The biopsychosocial model

stated that 'no single illness or person is reduced to any one aspect'. The psychodynamic and medical models assert that the quality of our social relationships has a major impact on our physiological systems, especially in terms of our ability to cope with stress and the end states of depression and anxiety. Evidence has been found which shows that the chronically stressed may be vulnerable to subtle forms of brain damage (Sapolsky, 1996), resulting in memory loss and compromised immune functioning.

Healthcare workers should consider the biological, psychological and social domains (see Figure 11.3) in assessing the patient and in devising strategies to promote their health and to use participatory and empathetic interactions to cultivate a trusting relationship.

Scenario 11.1

George is suffering from anxiety; he also has high blood pressure. When his care worker talked to him, he disclosed that he had a very stressful but lowly paid job, it paid just enough to cover his monthly bills. He said he ate a lot of junk food, high in salt, as he was too tired at the end of his day to cook properly. He also said that he didn't get out much and had few friends.

- Put George's disclosures into the model boxes:

Biological	Psychological	Social

- What advice would you give to George to reduce his anxiety and to help reduce his blood pressure?

Psychiatry

Psychiatry is a modernist approach, one that can trace its origins to the cultural transformations of the European Enlightenment and its quest to replace religious revelation with human reason as the path to truth and progress. Sigmund Freud (1856–1939) is considered the founder of psychiatry, although his work is considered contentious as it did not follow any scientific principles. The term was coined by Johann Christian Reil in 1808, from the Greek meaning 'treatment of the soul'. Qualified psychiatrists are trained as physicians who then undertake postgraduate training to become psychiatrists. Patients are treated by taking a case history and a physical examination to determine if there is a biological cause for the illness. Recent research using MRI scanners and new discoveries in genomics and neuroscience is finding biological markers that underpin disorders once understood as failures in brain circuit processing. Care workers undertake mental health assessments which assesses things such as the patient's speech, mood, phobias and obsessions, and abnormal experiences and beliefs as a way of aiding diagnosis and treatment.

Psychiatric treatment consists of drug therapy and psychological interventions, very occasionally surgical intervention (tumours, epilepsy) or electro-convulsive therapy.

Psychiatry has a mixed press, mainly due to its relationship with mental health legislation and the ability to 'section' people. Sectioning is the use of the various sections of the Mental Health Act 1983 (updated 2008) to place sufferers in secure accommodation and the enforcement of pharmacologic treatment regimens (Community Treatment Orders). In the same way that physicians can confuse patients with use of diagnostic professional language, so can psychiatrists and psychiatric assessments, using language that is difficult to understand and that exploits the power differential between the doctor and patient.

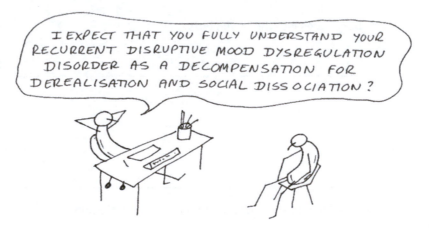

Figure 11.4   Power differential in psychotherapy

Jerome Frank (1961) surveyed the world of psychotherapy. He came to the conclusion that all forms of therapy, even those with very different theoretical frameworks, worked on the basis of a common set of essential elements. These were:

- a helping relationship with a thoughtful and concerned listener,
- a clearly defined space in which healing could take place and
- the use of some 'ritual' which served to strengthen the relationship between therapist and client.

📺 Scenario 11.2

Robert is a retained firefighter, this means he carries an alerter when he is at his full-time employment. When the alert goes off, he jumps in his car and drives to the fire station. This 'shout' is to attend a road traffic incident, where a car had hit a motorcyclist. The rider was missing when the crew arrived at the scene. Robert found the rider's body in a hedge. The force of the collision had taken the rider's legs off. The firefighters worked with the ambulance crew and the police. When the scene was cleared, Robert returned to work. A few weeks later, Robert began to have nightmares always leading to images of the rider. To help him sleep Robert began drinking heavily, and when his wife challenged him on this, he lashed out and hit her. The following day he was deeply ashamed of his actions and sought help. What diagnosis would you suggest and what therapy might help him?

MENTAL HEALTH AND STIGMA

As explained earlier, whether a behaviour is considered normal or abnormal depends on the context and culture surrounding it. Archaeologists have found 7,000-year-old skulls with holes drilled into them, no one really knows why but the current explanation is either to relieve headaches or to let demons out (possibly epilepsy). The ancient Greeks blamed the uterus (in women) and called it hysteria. In early medieval times, possession by the devil was the prevailing view and women were blamed and burned as witches. By the sixteenth century, asylums were established to contain the mentally ill and quite often these were seen as a source of entertainment. People went to places such as St Mary of Bethlehem in London (which gave us the name Bedlam) to watch the crazy people.

Asylums were generally overcrowded and custodial in nature. The rise of the age of Enlightenment in the late eighteenth century led to a different explanation, that of the medical model and the disease process, although many still felt that mental ailments were the products of moral defects in the character. In 1883, the German psychiatrist Emil Kräpelin (1856–1926) developed a naming system of psychological disorders that consisted of a grouping of symptoms. Kräpelin described what he called 'dementia praecox', which is now better understood as schizophrenia.

People throughout history have been stigmatised for being mentally ill and this is still true today. Social stigma considers that people are uncomfortable with people who are unwell. They are viewed as 'abnormal', in fact we still study 'abnormal' psychology. Such people are different and they may be dangerous, they may behave in unexpected ways or be violent, therefore they are not to be trusted and should be treated with caution. The perpetuation of this view, especially through the media, can lead to self-stigmatisation. When the sufferer internalises stigma, this can significantly affect feelings of shame and lead to poorer treatment outcomes and increased social exclusion. Research by Livingstone and Boyd (2010) found that 'internalised stigma was positively associated with psychiatric symptom severity and negatively associated with treatment adherence'; this was especially true when researchers examined self-stigma in schizophrenia (Kung et al., 2008).

Labelling theory

Society determines which behaviours are non-deviant and deviant; behaviours that do not fit with social expectations are labelled deviant. The consequences of being labelled as deviant can be far-reaching and have an impact on the labelled person's self-belief systems. Some choose deviancy (criminals), adolescents quite often go through a deviant phase (delinquency: Sykes and Mazda, 1957; Matza, 1964) and some have deviancy thrust upon them. People suffering poor mental health fall into the last description. Sociologists would explain that deviancy definitions are framed by the powerful and wealthy (judges, politicians, medical professionals) generally against the poor or marginalised and that they make the rules that define the context of deviant behaviour. An examination of prison populations showed that more than 70% of prisoners have two or more mental health disorders. Male prisoners are 14 times more likely to have two or more disorders than men in general, and female prisoners 35 times more likely than women in general (Social Exclusion Unit, 2004). Lord Bradley's (2009) review of mental health and learning disabilities within the criminal justice system said that 'there are now more people with mental health problems in prison than ever before. While public protection remains the priority ... custody can exacerbate mental ill health, heighten vulnerability and increase the risk of self-harm and suicide.'

Both Becker (1963) and Lemart (1967) examined notions of deviancy and they discussed the reaction of others in the explanation of deviance, and considered that 'secondary deviancy' impacts on those labelled deviant. It is in response to this labelling that the person changes their behaviour in accordance with the label, so the label becomes a 'self-fulfilling prophecy'. Diagnosis by a medical professional can offer a person an explanation of the symptoms they are experiencing but the person's behaviour may reflect their internal understanding of what the diagnosis might mean. Goffman (1968) suggested that the label (diagnosis) can 'spoil the sufferer's identity'. Goffman called the social reaction to the diagnosis 'an enacted stigma' and the person's internal reaction 'felt stigma' (now called self-stigma). Diagnosis is not value neutral; some diagnoses such as depression or anxiety carry less stigma, whereas schizophrenia is value laden.

Link and Phelan (2001) describe five components of stigma: labelling, stereotyping, separation, status loss and discrimination within the context of power differential. They consider status loss and discrimination occur when the stigma interferes with a person's ability to participate fully in the social and economic life of her/his community, although Goffman considers that the discrimination can ripple out beyond the sufferer to their family and friendship networks (he called this courtesy stigma) and that these networks are tainted by association. This can further impact on the sufferer's self-belief by adding guilt to the mix.

The Mind/Time to Change Alliance carries out an annual survey on attitudes to mental health, which shows that people are becoming more tolerant and understanding of people with mental health issues but the last survey (2015) shows that people still feel unable to discuss poor mental health or mental health ailments with their employer as they fear repercussions for their career. Also striking was the number of people surveyed who considered those with poor mental health as 'likely to be violent', whereas the reality is that mentally ill people are more likely to be themselves victims of violence.

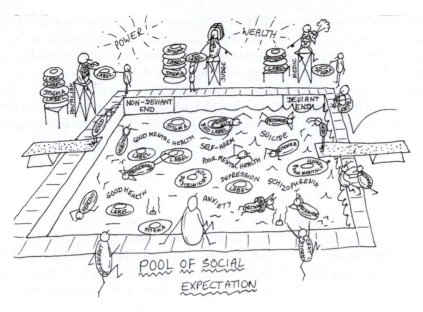

Figure 11.5   Pool of social expectation

Intersectionality in mental health

This discourse considers the effects of oppression on those with intersecting social, cultural and disabled identities. In the 1980s, Crenshaw and bell hooks opened a debate on black feminism and went on to develop a theoretical framework which brought together feminism and race to do away with the notion that feminism is a white enterprise, and that racial inequality and gender inequality are sides of the same coin. The debate has now widened to include all those who are marginalised by society for reasons such as gender, race, class, ability, sexual orientation, religion, caste, age and nationality. Intersectionality considers how such things can impact and interact on multiple levels, and the intersection perspective looks at the different types of discrimination (such as ageism, gender phobia, racism and bigotry) that an individual can suffer. Johnella Butler (2014) considers it is not just a quest for equality but a fight against injustice.

Seng et al. (2012) researched health disparities in post-traumatic stress syndrome and discovered that those with higher numbers of marginalised identities suffered from frequent discrimination leading to poor mental health. The social determinants of health play a major role in health and can compound health outcomes; those with multiple disparities can fall through the health support networks and this has cumulative effects on health.

TREATMENTS AND INTERVENTIONS

The medical model supports pharmacological interventions, but this has led to accusations that this is the only available option (the 'one trick pony' theory) and some consider the relationship between the medical model and the pharmacological industry corrupt. There is a belief that the pharmacological industry is engaged in 'disease mongering' or constructing novel diseases to create new markets for commercially available drug treatments. This debate is typified by the notion that high cholesterol, which was once an indicator of disease, has now become a disease in itself. This debate was at its most vociferous during the creation of DSM 5, when it was revealed that two-thirds of the psychiatrists compiling the manual had a financial relationship with drug companies (Cosgrove and Krimsky, 2012).

The pharmacologic revolution

The first recognisable drugs to be used in mental health treatment were sedative, hypnotic and anticonvulsive – potassium bromide, chloral hydrate (1830) and paraldehyde (1880). The first barbiturate was veronal (1903). The first major psychotropic drugs were the neuroleptic (antipsychotics) group, phenothiazines (tranquillisers), which became available in the early 1950s. This was considered the beginning of the 'pharmacologic revolution'.

Quite a few of the drugs prescribed for complex mental health conditions have unpleasant side effects, which is problematic for patients who have to balance using the drugs to control the ailment and living with the side effects. Many drugs can be given as a depot injection for those whose lives are too chaotic to take tablets or as a means of ensuring that medication is taken as part of a Community Treatment Order.

Schizophrenics are sometimes prescribed the drug Depixol (flupentixol), which in some people can lead to unwanted physical movements and facial tics, the so called 'Depixol dance'. Depixol is also addictive and needs careful management.

Quite a few antipsychotics can be toxic when taken with alcohol and some patients prefer to self-medicate using alcohol and street drugs. This leads to accusations of non-compliance and the use of legally enforced medication.

Interventions

Surgical intervention for psychiatric disorders is legal under the Mental Health (Treatment and Care) Act 1994 Section 70 (1). Psychiatric neurosurgery includes frontal lobotomy and ablation of the basal ganglia. The pathways involved in psychiatric illness are poorly defined and surgical results are variable therefore the practice of psychiatric neurosurgery has often been surrounded by controversy. Current practice tends to focus on the relief of symptoms such as epilepsy and Parkinson's disease, and it should be pointed out that fewer than 50 such operations take place each year (in the USA and UK). Electroconvulsive therapy has had a mixed press, although evidence suggests that it can help with severe depression.

The social model supports the various 'talking therapies', which include psychotherapy, psychoanalysis, counselling, cognitive behavioural therapy (CBT), acceptance and commitment therapy (ACT), neuro-linguistic programming, dance and movement therapy, eye movement and desensitisation and reprocessing therapy (EMDR), assisted animal therapy, hypnotherapy and latterly nutrition therapy. There are many complementary therapies, which include (but are not limited to) aromatherapy, anthroposophy, Ayurvedic medicine, Bach Flower remedies, healing and touch therapies, homeopathy, hypnotherapy, massage, naturopathy, nutritional therapy, reflexology, traditional Chinese herbal medicine, transcendental meditation and yoga, herbal medicine (Western).

Mental health support organisations offer such things as 'art for health' and 'walking for health'. Public Health England published a report (2016) which evidenced the benefits of art and exercise on health, and recent research by Frühauf et al. (2016) evidenced that exercise in the fresh air, even a short walk, had measurable benefit for someone suffering depression. Interestingly, the game Pokémon Go! is encouraging people to walk and sufferers of poor mental health have stated that playing the game is getting them out and meeting people. Leigh Alexander, writing in *The Guardian* newspaper, has said 'that mental health sufferers are encouraged to go out and interact' (Guardianonline, 19 July 2016).

Evidence-based practice

How do we know when we plan an intervention that it will work? Generally speaking, drug therapy has been through a rigorous process of testing before the drug comes to the market. Testing drugs for toxicity is a long process before it even gets to trials in human test subjects and costs run into several million pounds. Using animals in drug testing is contentious, as many feel this is cruel to the animal and that animal tissue does not respond in the same way human tissue does and therefore has little bearing on the effect the drug might have on people. The Draize eye test on rabbits has fortunately been replaced by more humane methods.

A key resource for evidence-based practice is the Cochrane Library, which offers high-quality, independent evidence to inform healthcare decisions. It holds six data bases of research documents and the library is used to conduct meta-analyses of research reviews. Cochrane Reviews are systematic reviews of research in healthcare and the data base (known as the CDSR) offers five types of review: intervention assessment, diagnostic test reliability, methodology reviews, qualitative reviews and prognosis reviews. The information generated can be used to influence practice, however, quite often best practice initiatives depend on healthcare professionals maintaining their CPD and searching out the best available evidence and finding means to implement them into their practice, not always an easy task, especially if funding is required.

MENTAL HEALTH IN A MULTICULTURAL SOCIETY

The cultural narrative explanation of mental health as formulated and categorised in the DSM reflects the normative values of America/Western Europe; however, this is not the world and different cultures have other explanations. Many early civilisations and societies were not literate and oral traditions were handed down by professional 'historians' or storytellers. The diaspora due to slavery or the genocide of Indigenous peoples by colonial invaders and settlers destroyed this repository of knowledge and forced a new Cartesian explanation of madness onto societies that had had a spiritual explanation.

The separation of mind and body

René Descartes (1596–1650) is considered 'the father' of modern Western philosophy. In his *Discourse on the Method and Principles of Philosophy* (1644) he states that he can prove his existence because he can think: '*cogito ergo sum*' – I think, therefore, I am.

In *The Description of the Human Body* (1648) he considered that the mind is separate from the body, suggesting that the body is a kind of machine, and this notion forms the basis of the biomedical paradigm because you can remove significant portions of the body but the mind remains intact. This idea of the two separate entities (Cartesian dualism) is central to modern Western medicine.

Societies that explain ailments in a whole body format (as opposed to dualistic) are now called 'holistic' and this is termed a 'metaphor', meaning a thing that is regarded as symbolic of something else. The term 'holistic' is applied to therapies such as counselling or massage, which is not its true meaning at all. Holistic medicine examines the individual in terms of their place in time and space and how they interrelate with their environment. This often includes their spirituality and the ways this is expressed, performing rituals and their place in the relationship with their relevant gods or spirits. Holistic therapies look for 'soul health', the restoration of spiritual and moral wellbeing as the means to holistic health. Religious people take great comfort from their beliefs and perform rituals to enhance their relationship with their god. Whatever your own beliefs are, you need to respect other people's beliefs and support them to access their ministers when they need to.

Cultural imperialism and mental health

At the end of the nineteenth century, within British colonies in Asia a part of the colonial medical officer's duties was to set up and run asylums. It was noticed that inmates who were judged mad smoked cannabis, and the British, being unaware that smoking cannabis was a normal social activity, determined that smoking cannabis made people insane (Mills, 2000).

At that time, very few non-Western countries used incarceration as a therapeutic intervention. In many rural areas, ritual, chants, herbal remedies, exorcisms and prayer was (and to some extent, still is) the normal healing practice. Some tribes welcomed those who heard voices, as they had clearly been chosen by the gods to become a shaman, the voice hearer, and their family were esteemed by the tribe. The Yoruba tribe in western Nigeria still practise traditional healing and pass on to trainees their knowledge verbally. Interestingly, the knowledge that they pass on is what works, and so it is continually updated through practical experience, an example of good evidence-based practice (Fernando, 2014).

MENTAL HEALTH FIRST AID

This programme was developed in Australia in 2000 by Betty Kitchener and Anthony Jorm and exported globally. It was adopted and launched in the UK by the Department of Health in 2007, and various organisations run training programmes for different sectors, organisations and communities, including the armed forces and youth leaders, in how to spot the signs of developing poor mental health and how to support someone evidencing the signs. It considers depression, anxiety problems, psychosis and substance use problems.

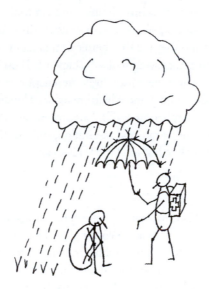

Figure 11.6   Mental Health First Aid

Would you know how to recognise the symptoms of someone becoming unwell?

- An unusually sad or irritable mood that does not go away
- Loss of enjoyment and interest in activities that used to be enjoyable
- Lack of energy and tiredness
- Feeling worthless or feeling guilty when the person is not at fault
- Thinking about death a lot or wishing they were dead
- Difficulty concentrating or making decisions
- Moving more slowly or, sometimes, becoming agitated and unable to settle
- Having sleeping difficulties or, sometimes, sleeping too much
- Loss of interest in food or, sometimes, eating too much. Changes in eating habits may lead to either loss of weight or putting on weight.

These are the classic symptoms of clinical depression (MHFA, 2008).

MENTAL WELLBEING AND RESILIENCE FOR YOURSELF AND THE PEOPLE YOU CARE FOR

Research suggests that there are a number of variables that make a far greater contribution to happiness than external and superficial factors, such as wealth and possessions. Biology has an important role in developing depression.

The role of neurotransmitters and mental health

Biologists would say only two things make you happy: dopamine (low amounts can produce anxiety and it has a relationship with schizophrenia) and serotonin (too little leads to depression, problems with anger control, obsessive–compulsive disorder, and suicidal ideation). These are neurotransmitters and they are the chemicals that allow the transmission of signals from one neurone to the next across synapses (see Chapter 5, Bioscience, for greater detail on the nervous system). Other neurotransmitters are norepinephrine and glutamate, which are important to the formation of memory and which are reduced by stress (which is why stressed students have difficulty in remembering stuff). Endorphins are involved in pain reduction and pleasure, these slow down heart rate and respiration, and GABA (gamma-aminobutyric acid) acts like a brake on adrenaline but too little leads to anxiety.

Resilience

When working for health, it is important to take care not just of the patients and clients in your care, but to take care of yourself. Working for health is a stressful undertaking; many things can impact on your own mental health such as worries, tiredness, workload, financial problems can drag you down too. Read the next few paragraphs on resilience and relate them to your own life and think about coping strategies that you can adopt to support yourself so you do not become overwhelmed and ill.

Seligman (2002) said that what distinguishes happy people from the unhappy is attitude, and that our attitude to our lives is determined by our character and genetics. He devised an equation to determine happiness:

H = Happiness

S = Set range (genetics)

C = Circumstances

V = Voluntary control (past, present, future)

- Past: Seligman says that when thinking about the past, people who are happy focus on good times rather than ruminating on the bad ones.
- Present: Seligman considers happy people take pleasure in their surroundings and their relationships and look for the good in each day.
- Future: Seligman says happy people are flexibly optimistic, they have a plan but are realistic in their goals and are not defeated if the plan doesn't pan out.

He also runs a website – www.authentichappiness.org – where you can take the 'happiness' tests.

Dr Timothy Sharp and colleagues (2013) have shown that identifying your personal strengths and qualities can lead to higher levels of happiness. However, they say that often people take the opposite course of identifying and then mending their weaknesses. Sharp et al.'s research suggests that focusing on strengths develops resilience.

Resilience is the capacity to cope with stress and adversity. Developing healthy coping mechanisms results in individuals bouncing back to a previous state of happiness, or using the experience of adversity to produce a hardening effect. Resilience is best understood as a process that promotes wellbeing or protects against being overwhelmed when in misfortune.

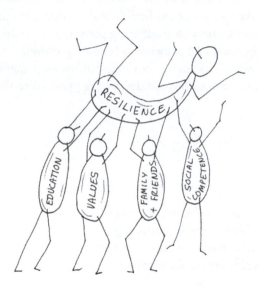

Figure 11.7   Resilience

Studies (Werner, 1970; Werner and Smith, 1992) show that the primary factor in resilience is having caring and supportive relationships within and outside the family. Relationships that create love and trust, provide role models, and offer encouragement and reassurance help bolster a person's resilience (Figure 11.7). Table 11.3 shows you what other factors can add to resilience.

Prepare for feeling overwhelmed and stressed by developing strategies that can reduce these feelings. Stress produces a somatic response as your body thinks you are

Table 11.3   Additional factors associated with resilience

The ability to make realistic plans and carry them out

A positive self-view and self confidence

Communication and problem-solving skills

The ability to manage strong emotions

under attack or in a frightening situation (fight or flight). The stress hormones cortisol and adrenaline need to be worked off and the best way to do this is to work with natural processes by taking exercise. Walking is free and you don't need any special training or clothing to do it; singing aloud to uplifting music and dancing will have the same effect.

CHAPTER SUMMARY

- This chapter has discussed notions of mental health. You have considered the various models of mental health and how mental health is categorised.
- The system of nomenclature of groups of symptoms by reference to the DSM and ICD has been explained, and this has shown that interpretations of which groups of symptoms make up a disease is flexible and changes over time.
- In order to help someone who is suffering poor mental health, you need to understand what can indicate that someone is becoming unwell. Understanding the way someone's behaviour is changing can help you to help them. Working for other people's health can tax your own, so developing personal resilience can support you in your role.

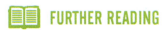 **FURTHER READING**

Websites

- Mind, the mental health charity: www.mind.org.uk
- Rethink Mental Illness: www.rethink.org
- Alzheimer's Society: www.alzheimers.org.uk
- Search on the NHS website for mental health: www.nhs.uk

Books and articles

All of these texts can support you in developing your understanding of mental health. You can read journal articles online and watch YouTube videos to deepen your knowledge:

- Frank, J. (1991) *Persuasion and Healing: A Comparative Study of Psychotherapy.* Baltimore: John Hopkins University Press.
- Gabe, J., Bury, M. and Elston, M. (2006) *Key Concepts in Medical Sociology.* London: Sage.
- Goffman, E. (1968) *Stigma: Notes on the Management of Spoiled Identity.* Englewood Cliffs, NJ: Prentice-Hall.
- Link, B. and Phelan, J. (2001) Conceptualizing stigma. *Annual Review of Sociology,* 27: 363–85.
- Seligman, M. (2002) *Authentic Happiness: Using the New Positive Psychology to Realise Your Potential for Lasting Fulfilment.* London: Simon and Schuster.

REFERENCES

Atkinson, R.C. and Shiffrin, R.M. (1968) Human memory: A proposed system and its control processes. In K.W. Spence, and J.T. Spence (eds), *The Psychology of Learning and Motivation* (Volume 2). New York: Academic Press. pp. 89–195.

Becker, H. (1963) *Outsiders.* New York: Simon and Schuster.

Bradley Report (2009) *Lord Bradley's Review of People with Mental Health Problems or Learning Disabilities in the Criminal Justice System.* Executive Summary. London: Department of Health.

Butler, J. (2014) *Leveraging Intersectionality: Seeing and Not Seeing.* Arizona: Richer Press.

Cosgrove, L. and Krimsky, S. (2012) A comparison of *DSM*-IV and *DSM*-5 panel members' financial associations with industry: a pernicious problem persists. *PLoS Medicone*, 9(3): e1001190. doi:10.1371/journal.pmed.1001190.

Engel, G. (1977) The need for a new medical model: a challenge for biomedicine. *Science*, 196: 129–36.

Fernando, S. (2014) *Mental Health Worldwide Culture, Globalization and Development.* Basingstoke: Palgrave Macmillan.

Foucault, M. (1973) *The Birth of the Clinic.* London: Taylor and Francis.

Frank, J. (1961) *Persuasion and Healing: A Comparative Study of Psychotherapy.* Baltimore: John Hopkins University Press.

Frühauf, A., Niedermeier, M., Elliott, L., Ledochowski, L., Marksteiner, J and Kopp, M. (2016) Acute effects of outdoor physical activity on affect and psychological well-being in depressed patients – A preliminary study. *Mental Health and Physical Activity.* Available at: www.science direct.com/science/journal/17552966 (accessed 14 March 2017).

Gabe, J., Bury, M. and Elston, M. (2006) *Key Concepts in Medical Sociology.* London: Sage.

Goffman, E. (1968) *Stigma: Notes on the Management of Spoiled Identity.* Englewood Cliffs, NJ: Prentice–Hall.

Goldacre, B. (2008) *Bad Science.* London: HarperCollins.

Illich, I. (1976) *Limits to Medicine: Medical Nemesis – The Expropriation of Health.* London: Boyers Publishing.

Kung, K., Tsang, H. and Corrigan, P. (2008) Self-stigma of people with schizophrenia as predictor of their adherence to psychosocial treatment. *Journal of Psychiatric Rehabilitation*, 32(2): 95–104.

Lang, R. (2001) *The development and critique of the social model of disability.* Paper given to The University of East Anglia. Available at: www.ucl.ac.uk/lc-ccr/lccstaff/raymond-lang/DEVELOPMMENT_AND_CRITIQUE_OF_THE_SOCIAL_MODEL_OF_D.pdf (accessed 10 April 2017).

Livingstone, J. and Boyd, J. (2010) Correlates and consequences of internalized stigma for people living with mental illness: a systematic review and meta-analysis. *Journal of Social Science Medicine*, 71(12): 2150–61.

Lemart, E. (1967) *Human Deviance, Social Problems, and Social Control.* London: Prentice Hall.

Link, B. and Phelan, J. (2001) Conceptualizing stigma. *Annual Review of Sociology*, 27: 363–85.

Matza, D. (1964) *Delinquency and Drift.* New York: Wiley.

McWilliams, N. (2009) Psychoanalysis. In I. Marini and M.A. Stebnicki (eds), *Professional Counsellor Desk Reference.* New York: Springer. pp. 289–300.

Mental Health Foundation (2017) *What is Mental Health?* Available at: www.mentalhealth.org.uk/your-mental-health/about-mental-health/what-mental-health (accessed 10 April 2017).

MHFA (Mental Health First Aid) (2008) *Depression Guidelines.* Available at: https://mhfa.com.au/resources/mental-health-first-aid-guidelines#mhfaesc (accessed 14 March 2017).

Mills, T.L. (2000) Depression, mental health, and psychological well-being among older African Americans: a selective review of the literature. *Perspectives*, 7: 93–104.

Mind and Time to Change (2015) *Latest Survey Shows Public are Less Likely to Discriminate against People with Mental Health Problems*. Available at: www.time-to-change.org.uk/news// latest-survey-shows-public-are-less-likely-discriminate-against-people-mental-health-problems (accessed 8 June 2017).

Parsons, T. (1951) *The Social System*. London: Routledge & Kegan Paul.

Public Health England (2016) *Arts for Health and Wellbeing: An Evaluation Framework*. Available at: www.gov.uk/government/uploads/system/uploads/attachment_data/file/496230/PHE_Arts_and_Health_Evaluation_FINAL.pdf (accessed 19 June 2017).

Robinson, M.D. and Gordon, K.H. (2011) Personality dynamics: insights from the personality social cognitive literature. *Journal of Personality Assessment*, 93: 161–76.

Sapolsky, R. (1996) Why stress is bad for your brain. *Journal of Science*, 9; 273(5276):749–50.

Seligman, M. (2002) *Authentic Happiness: Using the New Positive Psychology to Realise Your Potential for Lasting Fulfilment*. London: Simon and Schuster.

Seng, J.S., Lopez, W.D., Sperlich, M., Hamama, L. and Meldrum, C.D.R. (2012) Marginalized identities, discrimination burden, and mental health: Empirical exploration of an inter-personal-level approach to modelling intersectionality. *Journal of Social Science & Medicine*, 75(12): 2437–45.

Sharp, T., Moran, E., Kuhn, I. and Barclay, S. (2013) Do the elderly have a voice? Advance care planning discussions with frail and older individuals: A systematic literature review and narrative synthesis. *British Journal of General Practice*, 63(615): e657–e668.

Social Exclusion Unit (2004) *Mental Health and Social Exclusion*. Available at: www.nfao.org/Useful_Websites/MH_Social_Exclusion_report_summary.pdf (accessed 10 April 2017).

Sykes, G. and Mazda, S. (1957) Neutralization and Drift Theory. *American Sociological Review*, 22: 664–70.

Szasz, T. (1961) *The Myth of Mental Illness*. New York: Harper Collins.

Turbott, J. (1996) Religion, spirituality and psychiatry: conceptual, cultural and personal challenges. *Australian Journal of Psychiatry*, 30(6): 720–30.

Wakefield, J. and Horwitz, A. (2006) The epidemic in mental illness: clinical fact or survey artifact? *Contexts*, 5(1): 19–23.

Werner, E.E. and Smith, R.S. (1992) *Overcoming the Odds: High-risk Children from Birth to Adulthood*. Ithaca, NY: Cornell University Press.

Werner, J.A. (1970) To nursing practice. *Perspectives in Psychiatric Care*, 8: 248–61.

World Health Organization (2014) *Mental Health: A State of Well-being*. Available at: www.who.int/features/factfiles/mental_health/en/ (accessed 10 April 2017).

Zigmond, D. (2010) *The Medical Model—its Limitations and Alternatives*. Available at: www.marco-learningsystems.com/pages/david-zigmond/medical-model.htm (accessed 10 April 2017).

Zola, I.K. (1973) Pathways to the doctor – from person to patient. *Journal of Social Science Medicine*, 7(9): 677–89.

12

PROTECTING CHILDREN AND VULNERABLE ADULTS

Janette Barnes and Jade Carter-Bennett

For most parents, our children are everything to us: our hopes, our ambitions, our future. Our children are cherished and loved. But sadly, some children are not so fortunate. Some children's lives are different. Dreadfully different. Instead of the joy, warmth and security of normal family life, these children's lives are filled with risk, fear, and danger: and from what most of us would regard as the worst possible source – from the people closest to them.

Tony Blair (2003), Foreword to *Every Child Matters*

This chapter has been co-written by a social worker who has worked predominantly with children and by an adult social worker in order to give a holistic appreciation of the role of safeguarding across the life span. Janette discusses the assessment process involved in safeguarding children using the Every Child Matters/Helping Children Achieve (ECM/HCA) framework, while Jade discusses the No Secrets policy in adult social services, and discusses the use of advocates and the Mental Capacity Act 2005.

Glossary

- **Abuse** A form of maltreatment either by commission or omission
- **Advocacy** Someone who supports the client to ensure their rights are protected and asserted
- **Assessment** This could be of a developmental nature or a needs led survey

(Continued)

(Continued)

- **Child in need** Under Section 17 (10) of the Children Act 1989, a child who is unlikely to achieve or develop without the support of the local authority
- **Child protection** Supporting a child suffering, or likely to suffer, significant harm
- **Common Assessment Framework (CAF)** A standardised approach to conducting an assessment
- **Single Assessment Process** This is replacing the CAF, but the information collected is similar

INTRODUCTION

The quotation that opens this chapter comes at the beginning of the government's initial consultation document entitled *Every Child Matters* which was published in 2003 as a response to the findings of the Laming Report that same year after the death of Victoria Climbié. It lays out the nature of child protection. However, sadly, despite all best efforts to date, we still have children who are in dire need of help, support and protection. In March 2015, the number of children who were 'looked after' was nearly 70,000, a 1% increase from the previous year and 6% compared to 31 March 2011. Currently, the majority of those children are cared for by foster carers (Department for Education, 2015).

Alongside these concerning statistics for children, there have also been many cases of severe harm resulting in the death of vulnerable adults despite the *No Secrets* White Paper (Department of Health, 2002). Following the murder of Steven Hoskin, a man with a learning disability who lived alone and was tortured before his death in 2006, a serious case review in 2007 found that agencies including health, social care and police had missed signs that should have initiated adult protection procedures.

In this chapter, we hope to give you an insight into the five essential building blocks for children to develop and grow into well-balanced happy young adults. We will also look at different aspects covered in the assessment process used by local authorities' social services departments, and how these form a holistic mechanism to allow you and other practitioners to make reasoned judgements about safety and needs once in possession of the relevant information. We will also aim to give an insight into how this is relevant within Adult Social Services because it supports the identification of eligible social care needs in terms of ensuring every opportunity for support to parents is offered. This is explained later in the text, with reference to the Care Act 2014. Also, we show how local authorities can use toolkits such as the Signs of Safety model, originally created for 'keeping children safe' which has been adapted to identify and manage risks to vulnerable adults.

We will look at the importance of attachment; how this combined with structure and boundaries, and in addition to basic needs for care and love, fosters resilience, growth and development throughout childhood. You will note that we have focused most closely on the needs of the children; however, we will also look at the needs of parents in terms of support and guidance to ensure their children are safe and well looked after and how such support can impact their ability to effectively parent their children and keep them safe.

Go Further 12.1

Read the Children Act 1989/2004 (or see Working with Kids, 2017, for a good practical explanation) and other guidance and legislation, such as the Signs of Safety Model. Your knowledge and understanding of these will support your practice.

EVERY CHILD MATTERS/HELPING CHILDREN ACHIEVE

Every Child Matters (ECM) and its subsequent incarnation as *Helping Children Achieve* (HCA) sets out five aspects that should be addressed for all children so that they can have a safe and happy childhood wherever possible with their birth family. It covers all the things that a child needs to ensure their safety, development and happiness as they grow, and the aspects can be remembered with the acronym SHEEP.

Staying Safe: Protecting children from harm, neglect, or abuse while they are growing up; and equipping them with the skills for independence. There is lots of guidance and information around safeguarding children, but you need to know where to look. Activity 12.1 offers you some guidance.

⚙ Activity 12.1

What protocols does your own organisation follow and how will you contribute to this for the children and families you meet through your work?

Reflect on your current knowledge. Imagine a child discloses something untoward to you that will impact on their safety:

- What do you do?
- What are your organisation's procedures; do you know where this information is?
- Who can you talk to? And what is your moral obligation to the child?
- What are your observations – for example, home conditions, child's presentation, parent's actions/inactions? Consider how Bronfenbrenner's Systems Theory (1979) helps to explain how a child's development is affected by their environment:

  - Is it putting the child at risk/significant risk?
  - What can you do? (this may depend on your role and moral obligations)?
  - Who else can help? (other professionals, family, school, police)?

Doing nothing, if you have concerns, **is not an option**.

Staying <u>H</u>ealthy: Ensuring children have good physical, emotional and mental health by ensuring they have a healthy lifestyle. How will you know this?

When you are with a child, observe them for the following factors:

- Child's presentation – physically and mentally: are their appearance and reactions as you might expect? For example, injuries, stature, cleanliness, confidence, eye contact.
- How does the child interact/react with parent/s or primary caregiver?
- How does the child interact with others? Confident, quiet, withdrawn, fearful?

Doing nothing, if you have concerns, **is not an option**.

<u>E</u>njoying and achieving: As is their right, all children should be enabled to enjoy their lives and get the best out of it while achieving their potential for living independently. What can you do to help?

- Do parents help the child/ren to develop skills for future life?
- Are there opportunities for the child to socialise and learn from others?
- Is disability and support looked at positively?
- Do parents need support to help their children?

Doing nothing, if you have concerns, **is not an option**.

<u>E</u>conomic wellbeing/overcoming poverty: Overcoming their socioeconomic disadvantages to achieve their full potential in life.

- Do parents have knowledge of and access to universal and targeted benefits for the child?
- Housing – does this meet needs? If not how can this be addressed?
- Do parents keep the child safe, and give them a secure social structure in which to live and thrive?
- Is the child loved by family and friends, do they have continuity of love and support from principle caregivers – positive attachment and ultimately the basis for resilience? And does the child have self-esteem, confidence? Is the child able to achieve in life, education, social scenarios?

Yes, you guessed it – doing nothing **is not an option!**

Go Further 12.2

Maslow, A. (2014 [1962]) *Towards a Psychology of Being* (3rd edn). Bensenville, IL: Lushena Books. Read Essays 13 and 14 to deepen your knowledge.

<u>P</u>ositive contribution: Enabling children to make a positive contribution to their community and society, and not engaging in anti-social or offending behaviour.

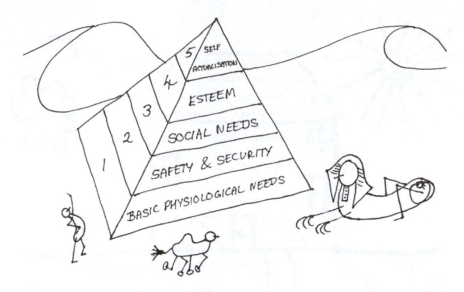

Figure 12.1   Maslow's pyramid of needs

What opportunities does the child have?

- Are disability or socioeconomic issues a barrier? If so how can this be overcome?
- What are the significant issues in the child's life preventing achievement?
- Does this relate to Maslow? Where is the gap in meeting lower level needs which inhibits self-actualisation?
- What can you do to help break barriers/enable needs to be met?

We will be taking a closer look at how these areas are assessed when a child and their family are facing difficulties. The failure of one or more of these areas being addressed may lead to difficulties in other areas, for example, un-addressed bullying of a child at school may lead to poor educational achievement and/or attendance, and increased friction at home, perhaps an escalation in unacceptable behaviours at home or in social settings. It is not always the case that the child is willing or able to articulate their fears or concerns and it is up to others – family, friends, school, GPs and others – including you – to help them by spotting the signs and symptoms, and ensure the right support is sought and put in place for them.

📖 Scenario 12.1   Amy

Amy is a seven-year-old child attending primary school and living with her mother, a single parent, in a two-bedroomed home in Newtown. They have recently moved to the area and Amy has been enrolled in school mid-term. The family do not know anyone in the local area; her grandparents live in another part of the country.

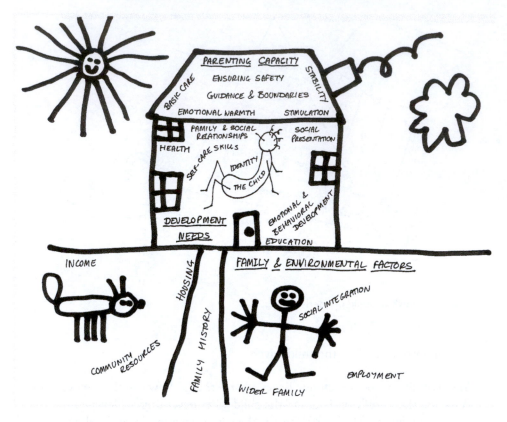

Figure 12.2   Assessment of children in need and family information.

© Alan Davidson, The Scottish Government, Better Life Chances Unit

For the past week Amy has been late on several occasions. She has been dressed in appropriate clothing but the clothing is dirty and she appears to have had only a minimal wash. She has been noted to be hungry, swooping on food at lunch-break and taking crisps and biscuits from the children who bring packed lunches. When challenged about this she says she is hungry because she did not eat her breakfast. She appears wary and does not make eye contact with her teacher, shunning other children who taunt her, calling her names, 'Smelly' and 'Piggy'.

Today, Amy arrives at school late, subdued and remains quiet all morning. Just before lunch she is excused to go to the toilet and when she returns to class just as the children are lining up to go to lunch, it becomes obvious that she has had an 'accident'. The class-room assistant takes Amy to one side, then to the school nurse, as it is apparent that the child is both embarrassed and in some discomfort. When the school nurse attempts to assist Amy, not only is it evident that she has soiled, but she also has some red blotches on her upper thighs which were noticeable when she lifted her dress.

What happens next ...?

Think about your organisation's protocols and relevant legislation or if you are not working in a child environment, think about what you would do if a friend was telling you this scenario, what advice would you give her/him?

Think about the children and young people you know in your professional or private lives. How might you notice the signs of need, or a child who needs protection? How might you play your part in dealing with this, or helping to ensure the need is met? How would you help Amy?

NO SECRETS: SAFEGUARDING VULNERABLE ADULTS

The *No Secrets* (2000) document is a government White Paper from the Department of Health which guides the development and implementation of policies and procedures to protect vulnerable adults from harm and abuse.

The guidance includes the broad definition of a 'vulnerable adult' as a person 'who is or may be in need of community care services by reason of mental or other disability, age or illness; and who is or may be unable to take care of him or herself, or unable to protect him or herself against significant harm or exploitation'. The *No Secrets* guidance details the different forms of abuse as physical, sexual, psychological, financial, neglect and discriminatory. Table 12.1 asks if you have the knowledge and understanding to intervene if you suspect abuse.

Table 12.1   Remember: abuse can take place anywhere

1. What do you do if you suspect abuse is occurring? As described previously, this may depend on your role. However, doing nothing is not an option.
2. Are you familiar with your organisation's Adult Safeguarding policy? You need to ensure you know what process to follow.
3. Who can help? Consider your line manager, police, CQC, Adult Safeguarding department of your local authority or if you are on placement and at college, your college safeguarding team can signpost you.
4. Consider mental capacity under the Mental Capacity Act 2005. This is particularly relevant as informed consent may inform your intervention. Advocacy is also important to this – this is mentioned in more detail later in this chapter.

Think about adults you have met both professionally and personally. Would you recognise the different forms of abuse as detailed in the *No Secrets* guidance? What would you do next? What evidence is there to inform your intervention? Read the case study in Scenario 12.2 and consider how you would react. We all have a part to play in ensuring the safety and prevention of harm to adults. Safeguarding adults includes the responsibility of supporting people to make informed choices and having control of their lives. In health and social care, there are principles set out that are agreed within the Care Act 2014 that help us to understand how to safeguard adults, particularly those who are considered vulnerable. These are:

[1] Empowerment: Ensuring people have all the information available to them in order to make their own decisions.
[2] Prevention: Taking preventative measures before harm can occur.

[3] Proportionality: The least restrictive or intrusive intervention to risk presented.
[4] Protection: Support, advocacy, representation.
[5] Partnership: Solutions through the exploration of services within the community.
[6] Accountability: Transparency and accountability within the practice of safeguarding.

Scenario 12.2   Mary

Mary is a 25-year-old woman with a learning disability. Mary lives with her mother and two siblings, who are also adults but do not have learning disabilities. Mary is currently pregnant with her first child. The relationship between her siblings and Mary is volatile, often resulting in verbal arguments.

Mary told her midwife that she currently sleeps on her mother's sofa due to her sibling moving into her bedroom and Children's Services are involved due to concerns around Mary's capacity to effectively and safely parent her child without support because of her own learning needs.

During a meeting, Mary presented as wearing weather-inappropriate clothing and stated that she did not have enough money to buy a coat. Mary went on to say that this was because she had given her mother money for the rent and she had needed to pay for the household weekly shop as her mother could not afford it.

● What types of abuse may be occurring here?
● What would you do next in supporting Mary to remain safe?

PROFESSIONAL STANDARDS: ETHICS, CONDUCT AND PERFORMANCE

Social Workers, Occupational Therapists, Teachers, Doctors and Nurses to name but a few are bound by guidance or a code of conduct, performance and ethical standards. For example, as Social Workers our registration is with the Health and Care Professionals Council (HCPC). Thus we are committed to ensuring that we 'promote and protect the interests of service users and carers', we must 'communicate appropriately and effectively', 'work within the limits of my knowledge', 'delegate appropriately', 'respect confidentiality', 'manage risk to self and others', 'report concerns about safety', 'be open when things go wrong', 'be honest and trustworthy', 'keep records of our work' (HCPC, 2016).

The evolution of policies, legislation and guidance has meant that professional development is at the forefront of social work, ensuring the continuous updating of knowledge so that the HCPC standards can be consistently adhered to. Perhaps the most common of these knowledge frameworks is the Professional Capabilities Framework, developed by the Social Work Reform Board. This standards framework sets out the expectations of social workers at each career stage. Many employer organisations also have their own professional development systems which promote and support performance of the professionals within it. For more information about ethical codes, read Chapter 2, Values and Ethical Frameworks in Health and Social Care.

ASSESSMENT, SUPPORT AND ADVOCACY

Assessment of needs: children

When concerns are raised about a child to the local authority, either by an individual or an organisation, the local authority has a duty to make enquiries, and take whatever action to consider whether the child is a child in need or a child at risk, as described in the Children Act 1989/2004.

You will always have someone in your organisation that you can share concerns with and seek guidance from, and there is likely to be a delegated person who will ensure the local authority are informed. One of the most important things you should do is to ensure you make an accurate record of your concerns, of anything that a child discloses to you, and then take it to the appropriate person. This will enable social services to make their enquiries and assess needs if this is necessary.

Since April 2014, the system of assessment changed to a Single Assessment Framework and this replaced the Common Assessment Framework (CAF) and the Children in Need (CIN) assessment. (Local authorities will have different formats for collecting the information but they will all cover the same information.) The 'My World Triangle' details child-centred factors for consideration when writing an assessment (see Figure 12.3).

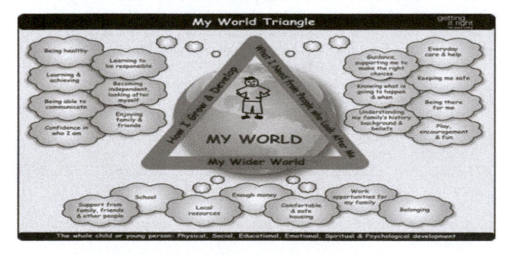

Figure 12.3 My World Triangle

© Scottish Government Better Life Chances Unit

Despite the change in name and perhaps format, the Single Assessment Process continues to maintain the principles that were enshrined in the Common Assessment Framework, that is, the holistic assessment of the child and family in order to determine needs and the systems/theories and strategies needed to protect and enhance children's lives. Wherever possible, this would be achieved with a child remaining in the care of their birth parents, when this can be done safely and in the child's best interests.

The Children Act 1989 states in Section 20 (or s.31, depending on which section of the Act you are applying) that where possible, required action should be taken without recourse to the courts. All assessments should have the child at its centre and should ensure that the child's voice is heard. It must, in addition to the needs of the child, assess the ability of the parents or main caregivers to parent the child successfully. In effect, the same areas as the CAF addressed should still be covered:

- The child's development needs
- Parenting capacity
- Environmental factors

 There is, rightly, great emphasis on the assessment allowing the child's voice to be heard throughout. The child's needs, and the risks they are or may be exposed to, have to be assessed and analysed alongside the child's own strengths, including their quality of attachment to parents. This is alongside their parents' strengths and resilience and the support they can call on from the wider family network. Equally, the protective factors need to be assessed – many families and parents would struggle without the help of others, be they extended family and friends, or professional support from schools, health and other professionals in the social care or healthcare system.

Although there is now a Single Assessment Process, there is also an Early Help Assessment which forms the initial part of that process and allows for essential help to be put in place as quickly as possible.

Here are the areas to be covered in the Single Assessment Process:
For the child:

[1] Health and the actions to ensure this is maintained – diet, exercise, physical and social stimulation.
[2] Learning and achieving – educational support and attainment, extracurricular activities and interests.
[3] Sense of self-confidence in who they are.
[4] A sense of their belonging and place within the family, extended family and their world.
[5] The child's social skills within the family and beyond.
[6] Self-care skills, and the child's level of independence.
[7] The support the child gets from family, friends and other significant people in their lives.

This assessment relies heavily on the skills of the assessor in engaging the child and establishing their feelings and wishes. It is important for all professionals working with the child to be honest and open with them. Many children lack the confidence and trust to talk to others about how they feel, and this may mean that the process of getting to know the child and the causes of their problems might be slow. This also might mean that the information you have, along with any evidence, including any disclosures made to you, is important to those carrying out an assessment.

It is important to ensure that your communication and actions support this process rather than inhibit it. Ensure you speak to children in a place that they feel comfortable, use language that they will understand and ensure they feel safe. Listening to the child is very important, as is clarifying information without leading the child's responses. It is very important not to ask any leading questions. Leading, which some might see as encouraging, might just get you what you want to hear and not necessarily what the child really wants to say/tell.

While there are occasions where children are removed from parents either immediately or after a period of time, there are many more children and parents who receive help and support from other sources in order to ensure their needs are met and they are deemed safe.

Assessment of needs: adults

The Joseph Roundtree Foundation (Dowling et al., 2006) explains, 'a move to outcome and needs based assessment would put the individual and their views, needs and wishes at the centre of the work, as the setting of outcomes is both a personal and subjective process.'

Every adult who appears to require care and support has a right to an assessment of their needs, regardless of their likely eligibility to receive state-funded care and support. The duties of the local authority in relation to assessing need are set out in the Care Act 2014, with a focus on how a person's needs can impact upon their wellbeing as well as what outcomes they wish to achieve.

When an assessment outcome results in an adult not being eligible for support, it is the local authority's duty to advise and signpost them in order to promote the prevention of further needs developing. One particular amendment to the way an assessment is carried out is the addition of caring for children as an eligible need. This has meant that it is considered an eligible need for support when someone's caring responsibilities are impacting on their wellbeing, and such needs going unmet. Assessing need of adults differs greatly to that of children; however one consistency is the role in safeguarding and identifying risk. Alongside need, safeguarding adults is paramount in adult services and it is important to know what to do when concerns arise. Concerns are often raised during the assessment process, which includes four specific outcomes:

[1] Managing nutrition. This includes the preparation of food and drink and the ability to eat and drink with or without support.
[2] Maintaining personal hygiene. This includes the ability to wash independently and manage the laundering of clothes.
[3] Practical aspects of daily living. This includes the ability to maintain a habitable home environment, making use of necessary facilities in the community, accessing and engaging in work, training, education or volunteering and caring responsibilities for a child(ren).

[4] Emotional wellbeing. This includes the ability to maintain and develop personal relationships, awareness and decision-making, and behaviours.

During the assessment process, it also important to consider the management of finances and what informal support is currently being provided. Also, included in the assessment is self-neglect. There are national guidelines available to determine the threshold for this. A key point during the assessment process is that of mental capacity, and ensuring that the adult has been given every opportunity to communicate their wishes whether capacity is determined or not. It is important that the service user is supported to ensure their views are central to the assessment process.

Advocacy

Advocacy is very important within adult services because it shapes the intervention, ensuring the service user's views remain central. Professionals must ensure that every adult receiving an assessment is offered advocacy to assist them in their decision-making process. Quite often, a person will have an informal carer, friend or relative who may be able to take on an advocacy role.

Independent advocates are required when someone is assessed as lacking the mental capacity to make a specific decision. This was introduced by the Mental Capacity Act 2005, which provides the legislation for safeguarding people who lack capacity. This includes decisions about where someone lives and about receiving medical treatment. It is vital that mental capacity assessments are decision- and time-specific, however capacity must always be assumed unless all steps have been taken to evidence otherwise. The five principles that underpin the Mental Capacity Act are set out in Table 12.2. There is also a duty for independent advocacy under the Care Act 2014 which means that local authorities have a duty to ensure people are involved in decisions about their care and support. Advocacy is required to support people in expressing their wishes and making decisions. More information can be found about advocacy within the Care Act 2014.

Table 12.2   Steps to capacity

1. The presumption of capacity
2. Individuals being supported to make their own decisions
3. The right to make unwise decisions
4. Best interests
5. The least restrictive option

Support for children and families

There is support for both children and their parents/primary carers. For example, there are a range of parenting programmes available for parents to support and enhance their parenting skills and resilience. This alone may be sufficient for the quality of parenting to be deemed 'good enough' after a period of monitoring. Support workers may be assigned to the family to help parents to establish routines and boundaries, help parents to build skills in communicating with their children, providing suitable stimulation, ensuring their health and safety, putting the child's needs at the centre of what they do. Equally they may need more specific support to help cope with issues such as disability or mental health needs (either the parent's or the child's). Health and social care professionals will work together to provide appropriate support.

Consider the models of multi-agency working, including the link into adult assessment for parents, support from mental health professionals, Education and Health Care Plans (EHCP), which run until a person is 25 years old and so cross the transition between children's and adult services.

Support for adults is not limited to parents however, with the implementation of personal budgets and direct payments for adults with eligible social care needs. This means that adults are now given the opportunity to choose and manage their own support should they wish to and have the mental capacity do so. Support is often to promote the safety of an individual and while meeting assessed unmet needs, encourages independence wherever possible. Much like children's services, a multi-agency approach may be needed to ensure effective outcomes when it comes to support. Examine the scenario below and think about the multi-agency response needed to protect and support this family.

💬 Scenario 12.3

A referral is received by social services from an anonymous source about a family of four living near Newtown. The information is that the house is plagued by mice and there is rotting rubbish in both front and back gardens as well as pieces of rotting furniture, including bed frames. The children who range from age 2 to 12 are often in the garden unsupervised and look dirty, dishevelled and undernourished. Sometimes even the youngest child is to be found playing in the street which, although not a main road, does have above-average through-flow of cars as it is used as a shortcut to bypass the town.

Initial enquiries reveal that the children are often dirty and hungry at school, and often off sick, with the youngest two children having continence problems. Although there are no serious health concerns recorded by the family doctor, it is discovered that the mother is supporting her children alone, is dependent on benefits, and has in the past had problems with anxiety and depression.

The referral was made because a known drug dealer has been seen going into the house several times recently and the referrer said they believed he was living there some of the time.

- Consider the family circumstances and list the different types of help they may need.
- Where do you think that help will come from?
- What action do you think is required?
- Who will deal with this?
- Support for both adults and children – how might this differ?

Transition from childhood to adulthood

Regardless of whether or not a child receives services from the local authority, if they are likely to have needs following their eighteenth birthday the Care Act 2014 states that the local authority must carry out an assessment. This includes transition assessments for children, young carers, those detained in the youth justice system and young people receiving mental health services. The Care Act 2014 as well as the Children and Families Act 2014 provide legal guidance for young people with support needs who are preparing for adulthood. This process involves collaborative working across agencies. A pivotal point within this process is that while the child's needs and wishes should be at the forefront of any intervention, once an adult they have a legal right to make their own decisions around their care and support. The Mental Capacity Act 2005 applies to individuals age 16 and over and is therefore a vital law during this transition process. The Act is explained in more detail earlier in this chapter.

ATTACHMENT THEORY

Attachment theory (Bowlby, 1951) considers that a strong emotional and physical attachment to at least one primary caregiver is critical to a child's personal development. (Further detail about attachment theory can be found in Chapter 8, Applied Health Sciences.)

We know from Bowlby's research that attachment develops from very early on in a child's life and that different types of attachments are formed (Ainsworth, 1974) and attachment shapes and affects a child's sense of self, and their relationship with others. The lack of secure attachment in early childhood, when left unaddressed, will set the pattern of action and reaction to caregivers in later life, and may inhibit the developing child from forming positive attachment to others, sometimes for the rest of their lives.

A good understanding of attachment theory and the behaviours that might ensue from different types of attachment is essential when working with children and families. Not only will there be issues for the child who does not have a secure attachment, but the inability to support that secure attachment may stem from the parent's inability to form secure and lasting attachments themselves. Their own childhood and development may have been shaped by a lack of secure attachment.

Attachment types:

[1] **Secure:** The positive attachment to a primary caregiver who is there for the child and supports them to grow and develop healthily, developing self-confidence in life. Children who have a secure attachment are likely to be more resilient and able to make positive attachments to others and use their positive experiences in childhood when they become parents themselves.

[2] **Avoidant:** A child demonstrating this type of attachment may be very compliant with a parent's requests and instructions in order to avoid being rejected. These

children don't want to appear needy or wanting attention as this leads to the parent being angry or resentful. They become self-reliant and independent, showing little reaction when separated from the parent. The parent is likely only to show a positive response when the child is well behaved and not in need of attention, being hostile and rejecting at other times.

[3] **Ambivalent:** Arises where the caregiver is inconsistent in caring for their child, and is neglectful through being unable to empathise with the child and their needs. The parent is likely to be responsive to the child more to meet their own need and not the child's. Children subject to this will both seek and reject parental attention and support, leaving them confused and with low self-esteem.

[4] **Disorganised:** This results from the parent or caregiver being angry, rejecting, or displaying behaviour that frightens the child. There is no emotional attachment or commitment and this is often linked to parental dependence on drugs, alcohol or other substances. Their own needs are of greater importance than the child's. The resultant anxious child may seek solace from the parent who has also been the initial cause of their anxiety. Children with disorganised attachment are often very disturbed, unable to form positive social relationships, and often display aggression that is difficult to address.

Many children in the care system will display evidence of insecure attachment of some kind. Hopefully with patience, support and therapeutic interventions, practised consistently, the child may be able to learn to form positive attachments with alternative caregivers and gain resilience and the ability to cope better with future life and its changes.

Attachment theory, from childhood to adulthood

Numerous studies suggest that it is infant attachment that is paramount in the shaping of personality and relationships, however there may be many challenges in adulthood as a result of an insecure attachment and it is argued that our primary caregivers can have a significant effect on this.

While this does not suggest that a child with poor attachment will be unable to create or maintain meaningful relationships or lead a fulfilling life, many studies have found that there are some developmental patterns typical of insecurely attached children. Bowlby's monotropic theory proposed the idea that a child's attachment type may be reflected in later relationships throughout their life. These challenges may include emotional detachment, fear of trusting relationships and confusing self-image as well as a lack of ability to manage complex and aggressive behaviours. By looking at the different attachment styles, we can hypothesise how this may impact a child as they approach and enter adulthood (see Table 12.3).

There is no clear 'treatment' for an adult who has experienced an insecure attachment as a child; however, it has been suggested that professional intervention may support and encourage an adult to learn to change behaviours over time, thus promoting

Table 12.3   Attachment in later life

Secure	An adult may be empathetic and be able to create and maintain meaningful relationships. A child who experiences a secure attachment may have more confidence in relationship building and creating boundaries.
Avoidant	As a result of a rejecting attachment or indeed an unavailable one, once an adult, the child may themselves be avoidant in close relationships, possibly intolerant and critical of others in the relationship. The child may learn to behave in such a way as to not appear to want attention and this may continue into later life.
Ambivalent	Due to the unpredictability of this attachment style, in that a parent is inconsistent in their caring role, this may lead to an adult being insecure and unpredictable in their relationships. Without having been given an opportunity to learn about meaningful relationships, future relationships may create anxiety and possible controlling behaviour.
Disorganised	Abusive relationships may result from a disorganised attachment and the child who experiences this type of attachment may become insensitive in later relationships during adulthood. This type of attachment can create fear in a child, which may lead to behaviours where it is felt acceptable by the adult to mimic the behaviours they experienced. Where a child who experiences this type of attachment may seek comfort from the caregiver who installs this fear, this may be a trait that is transferred into adulthood, meaning that the now adult may be at higher risk of abuse and/or neglect than an adult who had a secure attachment during childhood.

meaningful and fulfilling relationships throughout their life. If this intervention, be it through mental health, social or counselling services, is to be at its most effective, it is suggested that support is given at an earlier stage of an adult's life.

In addition to previously mentioned relationship behaviours, it is important to understand that this is not an exhaustive list of risks during adulthood and its transition, but rather an insight into how attachment theory may explain how relationships with others can be impacted upon. Studies show that children who do not experience a secure attachment are at higher risk of depression and substance misuse, however, there have also been studies that suggest these behaviours can be attributed to many other factors and may or may not put an adult at further risk of abuse or neglect. Preventative measures are key in reducing these risks.

CHAPTER SUMMARY

- We hope that you now understand the critical thinking and structure around identifying the holistic and specific needs of children, families and vulnerable adults.
- Children must have their basic needs met to a level where they can develop and enjoy life and reach their full potential, ensuring safety and promotion of independence for adults.

- You will understand the importance of listening to the child and ensuring their views are heard alongside assessing the skills and abilities of the primary caregivers, and how this is mirrored in adult services through the use of advocacy.
- You will also have an understanding of why mental capacity is so important and the legislation that underpins this.
- In addition to an understanding of your role and responsibilities around safeguarding children and adults in your care, you will have an appreciation of the many facets of the assessment process and your role in this, if any. You have looked at underlying theories, primarily attachment theory, and the importance of this to a child's development from conception onwards as well as the approaches within adult social care and how these often intertwine.
- This chapter would need to be a book on its own to give you all the answers and information available, but we hope it will give you food for thought and invite you to engage in further reading and research.

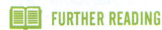 FURTHER READING

Relevant legislation and guidance

All of these can be found at www.legislation.gov.uk

- Children Act 1989
- Children and Families Act 2014
- Care Act 2014
- Mental Capacity Act 2005
- *No Secrets*: Guidance on protecting vulnerable adults in care (2000)
- *Framework for the Assessment of Children in Need and their Families* (2000)
- *Working Together to Safeguard Children* (updated 2017)

Books

These key texts will support your knowledge development and understanding of issues in working with children and families:

- Department for Education (DfE) (2013) *Working Together to Safeguard Children: A Guide to Inter-Agency Working to Safeguard and Promote the Welfare of Children (Safeguarding Children In Education)*. London: Shurville Publishing. Available at: www.gov.uk/government/publications/working-together-to-safeguard-children--2 (accessed 28 March 2017).
- Fowler, J. (2002) *A Practitioner's Tool for Child Protection and the Assessment of Parents*. London: Jessica Kingsley.
- Howe, D. (2011) *Attachment Across the Lifecourse: A Brief Introduction*. Basingstoke: Palgrave.

- Linden, J. and Webb, J. (2016) *Safeguarding and Child Protection: Linking Theory and Practice* (5th edn). London: Hodder Education.
- Maslow, A. (2014 [1962]) *Towards a Psychology of Being* (3rd edn). Bensenville: Lushena Books.
- Northway, R. and Jenkins, R. (2017) *Safeguarding Adults in Nursing Practice* (2nd edn) (Transforming Nursing Practice Series). London: Sage.
- Pitcher, D. (2014) *Inside Kinship Care: Understanding Family Dynamics and Providing Effective Support.* London: Jessica Kingsley.

REFERENCES

Blair, T. (2003) Foreword to *Every Child Matters*. Green Paper. Cm 5860. London: TSO.

Bowlby, J. (1951) *Maternal Care and Mental Health*. Geneva: World Health Organization Monograph.

Department for Education (2015) *Children Looked after in England Including Adoption: 2014 to 2015*. SFR34/2015 [online]. Available at: www.gov.uk/government/statistics/children-looked-after-in-england-including-adoption-2014-to-2015 (accessed 28 March 2017).

Department of Health (2000) *No Secrets: Guidance on Developing and Implementing Multi-agency Policies and Procedures to Protect Vulnerable Adults from Abuse*. London: DH.

Dowling, S., Manthorpe, J. and Crowley, S., in association with King, S., Raymond, V., Perez, W. and Weinstein, P. (2006) *Person-centred planning in Social Care*. Available at: www.jrf.org.uk/sites/default/files/jrf/migrated/files/9781859354803.pdf (accessed 10 April 2017).

HCPC (Health and Care Professions Council) (2016) *Standards of Conduct, Performance, and Ethics*. Available at: www.hcpc-uk.org/aboutregistration/standards/standardsofconductperformanceandethics/ (accessed 28 March 2017).

Laming Report (2003) *The Victoria Climbié Inquiry: Report by Lord Laming*. Cm 5730. London: TSO.

Working with Kids (2017) *Children Act 2004*. Available at: www.workingwithkids.co.uk/childrens-act.html (accessed 10 April 2017).

APPENDIX: NURSE ASSOCIATE DOMAINS AND WHERE THEY CAN BE FOUND

Domain	Chapter 1	Chapter 2	Chapter 3	Chapter 4	Chapter 5	Chapter 6	Chapter 7	Chapter 8	Chapter 9	Chapter 10	Chapter 11	Chapter 12
Domain 1												
Standards and values		√				√	√				√	√
Professional knowledge		√	√	√	√	√	√	√	√	√	√	√
Keeping up to date			√	√						√	√	√
Limits of competence/authority				√		√	√					√
How to seek support			√								√	√
Reflection on performance				√			√				√	√
Importance of personal integrity		√	√	√			√				√	√
Resilience and wellbeing			√	√			√				√	
The role of occupational health				√		√					√	
Personal strategies			√	√			√				√	
Importance of adhering to legislation, standards, policies, protocols and values		√		√		√	√			√	√	√
The importance of implementing health, safety and security policies						√	√			√	√	√
Report any actions or decisions which are not the best interests of any person in receipt of care		√					√			√	√	√
Promote evidence-based professional practice in person centred care			√				√				√	√
Act as a role model		√	√	√		√					√	√
Promote and exemplify safe and effective working		√		√		√	√			√	√	√
Domain 2												
The fundamental principles of nursing practice					√	√	√					
Describe the delivery of person-centred care		√					√			√	√	√
Describe the importance of gaining consent		√					√				√	
Explain the importance of giving people choices		√					√				√	√

(Continued)

(Continued)

Domain	Chapter 1	Chapter 2	Chapter 3	Chapter 4	Chapter 5	Chapter 6	Chapter 7	Chapter 8	Chapter 9	Chapter 10	Chapter 11	Chapter 12
Consider services from the family's point of view		√										√
Discuss concepts of choice, autonomy, empowerment, respect, holism, parity of esteem, empathy and compassion		√					√		√		√	
Consider changing plan of care to meet changing needs		√					√					
Support individuals to maintain their identity and self-esteem using person-centred values		√					√				√	√
Explain the impact of promoting effective health and wellbeing, empowering healthy lifestyles							√		√		√	√
Domain 3												
Describe the structure and functions of the human body					√	√				√		
Notions of health and ill-health (physical and mental)					√			√		√		
Societal impact								√	√	√		
Behaviour and lifestyle choices					√			√		√		
Genetics and genomics								√		√	√	
Disability					√		√			√	√	
Stage of life					√			√				
Socioeconomic factors and wider determinants of health								√	√	√		√
The impact of conditions on individuals, their families and/or carers										√	√	√
Reflect on how health behaviours impact on outcomes	√				√			√	√	√	√	
Population health and public health priorities						√		√	√	√		
Using physiological assessments and observations, in detecting and acting on early signs of deterioration							√					
Describe the role and practice of infection prevention and control and the potential signs of infection						√	√					
Individual's nutritional status and the ways this impacts on their overall health and condition	√				√		√				√	
Explain drug pathways and how medicines act							√					
Describe the impact of an individual's physiological state on drug responses and safety,							√				√	
Explain pharmacodynamics, the role of drugs and their mechanisms of action in the body							√					
Discuss medication in terms of risks versus benefits							√					
Describe the role and function of the bodies that regulate and ensure the safety and effectiveness of medicines					√		√					

Domain	Chapter 1	Chapter 2	Chapter 3	Chapter 4	Chapter 5	Chapter 6	Chapter 7	Chapter 8	Chapter 9	Chapter 10	Chapter 11	Chapter 12
Describe and discuss the management of adverse drug events,							√					
Explain the importance of consent with regard to administering medicines							√					
Describe individual legal responsibility, personal accountability and regulatory requirements							√					
Explain statutory requirements in relation to mental health,							√				√	
Describe and explain legislation that underpins practice relating to medicines,							√					
Explain the importance of the safe handling of medicines,							√					
Describe health promotion in the context of health inequalities,								√	√	√	√	√
Describe the genetic and genomic contribution to health and common disease												
Explain the need to manage and organise workloads and the role of prioritising the delivery of care		√					√			√		
Explain behaviour change concepts and skills in relation to health, wellbeing and self-care								√	√	√	√	√
Monitor and record nutritional status and discuss progress or change							√			√		
Administer medicines safely and in a timely manner							√					
Communicate and act on any concerns about or errors in the administering of medicines							√					
Work within legal and ethical frameworks that underpin safe medicines management							√					
Correctly and safely receive, store and dispose of medications							√					
Use up-to-date information on medicines management and work within local and national policy guidelines							√					
Use sound numeracy skills for medicines management, assessment, measuring, monitoring and recording						√	√					
Use sound literacy skills to record and document accurately interventions			√				√					
Work safely and effectively	√					√	√		√	√	√	√
Engage collaboratively with a range of people and agencies			√				√		√	√	√	√
Treat individuals with dignity, respecting their diversity, beliefs, culture, needs, values, privacy and preferences	√						√		√		√	√
Have the courage to challenge areas of concern	√		√			√	√			√		√

(Continued)

(Continued)

Domain	Chapter 1	Chapter 2	Chapter 3	Chapter 4	Chapter 5	Chapter 6	Chapter 7	Chapter 8	Chapter 9	Chapter 10	Chapter 11	Chapter 12
Be adaptable, reliable and consistent, show discretion, resilience and self-awareness and provide leadership		√					√		√		√	√
Promote and demonstrate a positive health and safety culture						√	√		√	√	√	√
Domain 4												
Explain the importance of clear and effective communication for person-centred care		√					√				√	√
Understand duty of care, candour, equality and diversity		√		√			√		√		√	√
Promote clear and effective communication	√	√	√			√	√					√
Overcome barriers to clear and effective communication	√	√					√			√	√	√
Impact on verbal and non-verbal communication	√		√				√			√		√
Describe legislative, policy and local requirements and ways of working with information and data		√		√			√		√			√
Understand when action required when concerns about accuracy, security and confidentiality		√		√		√	√					√
Communicate complex, sensitive information to a variety of health and care professionals		√					√			√	√	√
Respond appropriately to verbal and non-verbal communication	√						√			√		√
Promote and use appropriate digital and other technologies to support effective communication	√						√		√			√
Document nursing care in a comprehensive, timely, logical, accurate, clear and concise manner		√					√					
Promote effective communication using a range of techniques and technologies	√						√		√			√
Domain 5												
Describe the personal qualities required to develop leadership competencies				√								
Critically reflect on performance to identify their own personal qualities,		√	√	√			√					√
Explain the importance of working with others in teams and networks to deliver and improve services				√					√			√
Discuss models of leadership				√								
Describe the role of technological innovations in improving health outcomes for individuals,								√				
Critically examine the supervisory and leadership opportunities and roles				√								√
Explain the ways health and safety systems and policies can be developed, monitored, assessed				√			√					
Take a lead with peers and others where appropriate		√		√					√			√

Domain	Chapter 1	Chapter 2	Chapter 3	Chapter 4	Chapter 5	Chapter 6	Chapter 7	Chapter 8	Chapter 9	Chapter 10	Chapter 11	Chapter 12
Critically reflect on personal performance	√	√	√	√								
Work effectively with others in teams and/or networks to deliver and improve services, encouraging and valuing the contribution of all.				√							√	√
Contribute to and support quality improvement and productivity initiatives within the workplace,				√					√			
Use clinical governance processes to maintain and improve nursing practice and standards of healthcare		√		√			√					
Demonstrate team working and leadership skills in the provision of a healthy work environment		√	√	√								√
Actively encourage, and work within, a team environment, including multidisciplinary teams		√	√	√			√					√
Engage in continuous service improvement for better health outcomes		√	√	√					√			
Champion safe working practices and a culture that facilitates safety		√					√					√
Promote the contributions and co-production by individuals,		√							√			√
Domain 6												
Describe their duty of care and the ways they are able to take reasonable care to avoid acts		√		√			√					√
Describe their duty of candour and the ways this can be demonstrated in practice		√										√
Define harm and abuse and identify sources of support and guidance to inform appropriate action		√					√			√		√
Describe and critically discuss the importance of the basic rights and principles of dignity, equality, diversity, humanity and safeguarding		√								√		√
Describe the ways individuals can contribute to their own health and wellbeing										√	√	
Understand your duty of care, candour, cultural competence, equality and diversity		√					√		√			√
Challenge areas of concern using appropriate behaviours and communication methods		√		√			√					√
Recognise the signs of harm or abuse and act on this appropriately							√			√		√
Treat all individuals, carers and colleagues with dignity and respect for their diversity, beliefs, culture, needs, values, privacy		√		√			√			√	√	√
Safeguard and protect adults and children				√						√	√	√
Encourage and empower people to share in and shape decisions about their own treatment		√					√				√	√

(Continued)

(Continued)

Domain	Chapter 1	Chapter 2	Chapter 3	Chapter 4	Chapter 5	Chapter 6	Chapter 7	Chapter 8	Chapter 9	Chapter 10	Chapter 11	Chapter 12
Demonstrate respect, kindness, compassion and empathy for all individuals, carers and colleagues		√					√					√
Avoid making assumptions and recognise diversity and individual choice		√					√		√	√		
Domain 7												
Explain and critically discuss core theories of learning	√			√					√			√
Describe the importance of feedback and the range of methods for giving and receiving feedback	√											
Applying the skills of reflection to identify personal development needs		√	√	√			√					√
Acting as a self-motivated professional		√	√	√			√		√			
Contributing to a culture that values CPD in recognising strengths		√	√	√							√	
Act as a role model for ongoing learning and development of professional knowledge, skills and capabilities		√	√									√
Domain 8												
Explain the importance of research, innovation and audit in improving the quality of patient safety	√										√	
Understand governance and ethical frameworks		√		√		√	√		√			√
Use and engage with evidence-based practice			√			√	√				√	√
The role of statutory and advisory regulatory bodies,				√		√			√	√	√	
Apply critical analytical skills in a research/audit/service improvement context,	√								√			√
Demonstrate research awareness in evidence-based practice			√			√			√			

INDEX